KETO INTERMITTENT FASTING

COMPLETE BEGINNERS GUIDE

2 Manuscripts for Lose Weight and Stay Healthy thanks to Ketogenic Meals Prep, plus a Motivations to Reset Diet and Diabetes Prevention using Fasting Method

purposes and should thus be thought of as universal. As befitting its nature, it is presented without assurance regarding its prolonged validity or interim quality. Trademarks that are mentioned are done without written consent and can in no way be considered an endorsement from the trademark holder.

--- eBook 1 ---

INTERMITTENT

FASTING

BEGINNERS GUIDE FOR

WOMEN AND MEN

*A Complete Book for Effective
Weight Loss, with Exercises,
Motivational Habits, & Delicious
Recipes*

Table of content

--- eBook 2 ---

KETO MEAL

PREP

COOKBOOK

Beginners Ketogenic Diet

For Weight Loss

With Low-Carb Food

Table of Contents

Chapter 6: Tempting Lunchtime Choices397

Introduction

Congratulations and thank you for purchasing **Intermittent Fasting Beginners Guide for Women and Men**: <u>A Complete Book for Effective Weight Loss, with Exercises, Motivational Habits and Delicious Recipes</u>. With so many diet fads and meal planning guides available on the Internet today, finding a starting point for your own weight loss journey can be a daunting task. Choosing a path for weight loss is a lot more than just "eating right"—it's making positive changes to your lifestyle, adjusting your hormones in a natural way, and looking at how you eat, and how your body works, in a new light. This book aims to be a comprehensive guide to walk you through the ins and outs of intermittent fasting while also showing how it compares to similar weight loss plans, so that you may decide for yourself if it will be the safest, most comfortable plan for you.

Before you jump into this book, there is one key concept for you to keep in mind. Intermittent fasting is not a diet. Rather than monitoring what you eat, you'll be monitoring when you eat. Fasting is a unique and ancient practice, and a tried and try method for burning fat while gaining muscle. It can be used in tandem with almost any dietary restrictions. The chapters that follow will discuss the science behind this method, explore the various ways intermittent fasting can be practiced, and give you a snapshot of how it will affect you in your daily life.

There are a plethora of books and weight loss plans available today, so thank you again for choosing this one. Please enjoy, and should this plan work for you, please spread the word!

Chapter 1:

<u>The Science Behind Fasting</u>

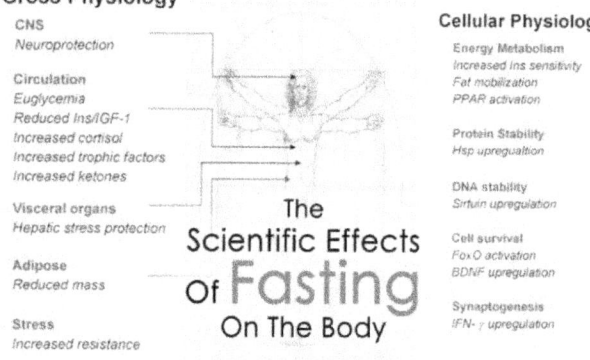

Gross Physiology

CNS
Neuroprotection

Circulation
Euglycemia
Reduced Ins/IGF-1
Increased cortisol
Increased trophic factors
Increased ketones

Visceral organs
Hepatic stress protection

Adipose
Reduced mass

Stress
Increased resistance

The
Scientific Effects
Of Fasting
On The Body

Cellular Physiology

Energy Metabolism
Increased Ins sensitivity
Fat mobilization
PPAR activation

Protein Stability
Hsp upregualtion

DNA stability
Sirtuin upregulation

Cell survival
FoxO activation
BDNF upregulation

Synaptogenesis
IFN-γ upregulation

Unlike a lot of modern weight loss plans, fasting is a lifestyle choice that is deeply rooted in the past and can be found throughout history. For as long as religion and scholars have existed, fasting has played a part in their rituals and cultures. Long before it was explored as a weight loss method, it was a discipline used to detoxify the body and mind, draw out core survival instincts, and bring mental clarity. And although it's advertised today as a method to burn fat fast, practitioners of intermittent fasting can still see the effects it has on their ability to sharpen their focus and reduce mental sluggishness.

Fasting: A Preparatory Stressor

Today, humans are wired to live much longer than we were in the past. With the external benefits of our modern world aside, we can thank our increasing longevity on our growing knowledge of biology and autophagy, hundreds of years of genetic trial and error, and a whole lot of exposure to physically stressful situations. That last bit may seem counterintuitive at a glance, but in the context of evolution, it makes more sense. As we have encountered and overcome—or succumbed to—the multitude of curveballs that life has thrown at us over the ages, our bodies and minds have remembered different ailments and dangers and revised themselves to be more prepared in the future.

When our bodies detect foreign or inconvenient stressors, even on a cellular level, they make adjustments to avoid or fix them. We adapt. Not all "stressors" are subjectively negative or harmful, but our biology is more objective than our minds, so stress is stress is stress. Disease and pain (like burns or broken bones) are stressors, but exercise is also a stressor. And naturally, hunger fits the bill as well.

If you've ever broken a bone, you've probably had a few people tell you that it'll be stronger and harder to break after it heals. Similarly, after you exercise vigorously for a set period, your muscles tear from the physical stress, often causing pain, tenderness, and temporary weakness. But as any gym-goer will tell you, you'll only get stronger or maintain strength as long as you're working out properly, not weaker. This strength is gained when your body repairs the tears in your muscles. In preparation for preventing future pain, your muscles get a little stronger after each regular repair.

Intermittent fasting is very similar to exercise in how it affects your cells. When your body detects repeated instances of prolonged hunger, as long as you don't give in to food cravings, it will begin to adapt accordingly. A few days into your fast, the gnawing feeling in your stomach will begin to subside. You may even feel fuller more quickly when it comes time to eat again. This is your stomach and various hormones adapting to your new eating style and learning when they need to start calling for more sustenance, instead of telling you when they're accustomed to being full. To that end, it is advisable t0 keep your intermittent fast on loosely the same schedule each day, so your body can more accurately adjust.

Another benefit of intermittent fasting as a preparatory stressor is that during the adjustment period, your body may rack up it's immunity to certain sicknesses, in preparation for the scenario where you aren't getting enough nutrients. Your cells don't know that you're basing your new eating habits around a schedule and plan; again, they're objective and desperately trying to keep you healthy. Intermittent fasting is a nifty way to "trick" your body into increasing your immune system.

Free Radicals & Oxidative Stress

One of the less popularly discussed causes of many different health and cellular issues is the release of free radicals. Free radicals are unstable molecules that are short-lived and highly reactive. The instability of free radicals is because the atoms have unpaired electrons, and consequentially, they actively seek out and bond with whatever other atoms happen to be around. Free radical production is a natural side effect of our metabolic processes, but many foods can severely increase the count, which is when the problems begin to arise. This is the major cause of oxidative stress, as well as many other severe health concerns.

Oxidative stress is the process of cellular degradation that, in addition to just generally damaging your cells, causes the effects of aging to occur much more rapidly. When free radicals are produced, they quickly look for other atoms to give or take electrons with. This can escalate to the exponential increase of free radicals, as more and more cells suddenly become unstable. The immediate symptoms that are usually signs of significant oxidative stress are brain fog, fatigue, noise sensitivity, and headaches. While these are all relatively common and temporary problems, oxidative stress is a very common issue as well —but with harmful long-term effects. Monitoring potential signs of oxidative stress and responding accordingly can be invaluable for reducing free radical production (and oxidative stress, by association) significantly in the future.

Impaired or weakened mitochondria are responsible for most of our natural free radical production. In addition to this, foods that are commonly classified as "inflammatory" also show a rapid increase in free radical creation.

Among the worst contributors are refined carbohydrates and sugars, certain vegetable oils, fats, and processed meat (like pepperoni and hot dogs).

The common issue between these foods is the amount of oxidization that they see before you ever consume them, making their free radical count much higher from the get-go. Many types of meat with added preservatives have a higher chance of being oxidized. Red meat, due to its high iron content, also becomes oxidized very easily. Fats and oils tend to oxidize when exposed to high temperatures, including deep frying. Additionally, the reuse of cooking fats and oils (like in the vats used to deep fry food) oxidizes them even more. If you've ever felt sluggish or irritable after a hearty meal of deep-fried meats, you can probably thank a whole lot of oxidative stress.

While oxidative stress is extremely serious, it isn't too difficult to keep in check. Eating foods that are high in antioxidants is an excellent, natural preventative measure. Green teas, blueberries, steamed vegetables, and nuts make up a very small sample of the dozens of delicious, antioxidant-rich foods that are easily incorporated into everyday meals. Antioxidants eliminate free radicals in our bodies by stabilizing the atoms' electrons, stopping them before they can spread into chains or cause cellular damage. Eating a salad or a handful of nuts each day can be a decent way to combat oxidative stress, even if you change nothing else about your eating routine. You'll read more about potential ways to incorporate antioxidants into your daily diet in **Chapter 4**.

Intermittent fasting also has many benefits that directly correlate to free radical reduction, so if you're worried about the amount of oxidative stress in your body, this is a great way to quickly reduce the effects— now and going forward. During an intermittent fast, your blood glucose drops in a way that first-time fasters probably haven't experienced too often. This forces your body to utilize other sources of energy, including fatty acids, to keep your cells going. Resorting to your fat reserves for energy kicks those nifty stressor-induced survival mechanisms into gear and helps your body dispose of poorly functioning cells in a powerful process known as autophagy. And when those poorly functioning cells go, so do the insufficient mitochondria that are over-producing free radicals.

Autophagy

Autophagy literally translates to "self-eating," and how it works is just as amusing. When your body is under a certain degree of physical or external stress, the process of autophagy begins. Your body's stronger cells send out a membrane, the autophagosome, to hunt down weaker cells and consume them. This plays a massive part in our overall health, energy, weight, and wellbeing. It goes hand in hand with fasting and advocates of intermittent fasting hail autophagy as one of the regimen's pinnacle benefits. You'll see the word pop up throughout the rest of the book, so let's get the specifics out of the before anything else.

While the literal (albeit minimally scientific) definition is fun to reiterate, autophagy is a biologic process that is invaluably important to your body. When that membrane finds cells to "consume," they are usually dying, weak, or ill. These insufficient parts are sent through your cells' lysosome, which recycles them back into your body as free fatty acids and amino acids, which are used as building blocks for new cells.

By breaking them down and putting the resulting molecules to use, your body is able to create stronger, more powerful cells while clearing out the unnecessary ones. Think of it as biology's inherent "survival of the fittest" mechanism. While you work to optimize your weight during your fast, your body is working on a cellular level to eliminate its weak links and strengthen you from the inside.

Recall reading in the previous section about how your muscles heal with more strength after you exercise. If you already guessed that the healing process of your muscles would be autophagy, you're correct! Simplistically put the process to look like this: exercise is a stressor which tears your muscles, resulting in damaged tissue and cells. This stressor triggers autophagy; the damaged cells are singled out and broken down, and the resulting energy is used to fortify the rest of the surrounding tissue.

Along with fortifying existing cells, autophagy can also assist in the regrowth of heart and brain cells. This adds an element of protection to your body's most vital organs. It promotes immunity and anti-aging effects, reducing the chances of deteriorating cell accumulations. On that front, although it isn't an end-all cure, autophagy has been strongly linked to protection against cancer, Alzheimer, heart disease, liver disease, and many other ailments related to cellular degradation and misfolded proteins.

Dr. Eric Berg DC, a chiropractor who utilizes nutritional education and natural methods to help his clients manage their weight, is a major advocate for the impact intermittent fasting has on autophagy. He has a variety of educational materials regarding autophagy on the Internet, including videos.

One of his focal points is that, along with clearing out weak and diseased cells, autophagy can also help rid your body of misfolded proteins. The accumulation of misfolded proteins can be a conduit for amyloid deposits, which have been linked to a number of neurodegenerative diseases. Alzheimer, Huntington, and Parkinson's diseases are a few you've certainly heard of, but the list of problems caused by amyloid deposits is lengthy. While amyloid deposits in the brain can result in Alzheimer and other diseases of that caliber, deposits are also found in the arteries of diabetic patients. Any malfunctions caused by amyloid deposits are generally referred to as "amyloid diseases."

Autophagy is absolutely invaluable in the prevention and management of amyloid-related diseases. Your lysosome—your cell's "garbage disposal," as Dr. Berg puts it—handles misfolded proteins in the same way it handles any other unneeded parts. It takes them in, breaks them down, and puts the resulting raw materials back into your body to be utilized.

Autophagy is a powerful tool that everyone's body inherently knows how to implement, and as with all of our automatic biological processes, researchers are consistently striving to find "new" ways to optimize its benefits. It is a comprehensive defense mechanism, immunity booster, anti-aging agent, and preventative method. Obesity, diabetes, cancer, and heart disease being are only a handful of examples of what autophagy fights against, because the way in which it cleanses your weakened cells and fortifies the stronger ones. Optimizing autophagy has the promising potential to help you nip any current or future internal ailments in the bud by cleansing and fighting against whatever may be causing them.

Beating Inflammation at Its Source

You have probably heard health advocates say "Inflammation is the root of all evil" before or some variation of the phrase. There are countless methods on the market for battling inflammation, and while many have fantastic anti-inflammatory benefits, it's hard to find one that counters inflammation as profoundly as intermittent fasting has proven to.

Inflammation can have extremely detrimental impacts on your quality of life. Severe, chronic inflammation can lead to a laundry list of life-long issues, including neurodegenerative diseases, arthritis, various chronic pain disorders, mental health issues... the list goes on. The short-term issues are equally impairing, including muscle and joint pain, irritability, brain fog, and general sluggishness or discomfort. The general consensus among medical experts (and those who suffer from chronic inflammation) is that there are no good side effects to inducing inflammation.

With its onset (such as after you eat excessive inflammatory foods), your body temperature may rise, and your energy will drop significantly. This is popularly referred to as a "food coma," which shows how often people acknowledge a general decline in activity post-eating. After a thanksgiving feast or a Superbowl binge, you aren't exactly functioning at your peak performance. With your insulin and organs working overtime to process how many carbs and sugar you've just gorged on, the rest of your body starts to slow down.

Autophagy is one way that fasting helps fight inflammation.

Since damaged cells promote inflammation, that thorough cleansing of weak, unnecessary cells is a great preventative method. It can also help eliminate free radicals, and by proxy, oxidative stress. But autophagy isn't the only weapon intermittent fasting brings in against the issue.

Intermittent fasting also has incredible benefits for increasing your insulin sensitivity. If you start becoming resistant to insult, this leaves glucose (sugar) building up in your blood until it's eventually put away as fat. Both fat accumulation and sugar—especially sugar—are almost always accompanied by noticeable inflammation. Sweet as it is, sugar is one of the worst villains in the world of inflammatory foods. And if it is allowed to build up in your body, unused, the increase in inflammation you experience will be astounding.

By increasing your insulin sensitivity, your body can more easily use glucose for its intended purpose, rather than stockpiling it for "later use." Insulin allows your cells to take in glucose and use it as one of your body's main fuel sources. By extension, increasing your insulin sensitivity not only reduces the amount of glucose building up in your system (and therefore, inflammation) but also gives you more vital energy.

Intermittent Fasting for Improved Cognitive Function

Here's a common situation: a while after your last big meal, your stomach begins talking. Loudly. After a while of listening to its growl, you might feel lightheaded and shaky—issues usually associated with low blood sugar. You might also feel excessively irritable, tired, or confused.

If that sounds familiar, you might be skeptical about this aspect of fasting. How could something like hunger improve mental clarity?

Think about it this way. As we look further back in history, our ancestors had less and less ease of access to food sources. Before any nutritional modernizations that we're familiar with today were implemented, ancient peoples were hunters, gatherers, and scavengers. Finding their next meal was consistently challenging. Yet somehow, their ability to survive, fight, and find new food sources wasn't compromised by gnawing hunger and low blood sugar. This may be something we can only infer since we weren't there—but studies have shown that death by starvation is pretty detrimental to reproduction and cultural longevity.

The general conclusion we can reach based on our ancestors' survival is that not eating 3 square meals a day isn't the worst thing in the world, and it can even be beneficial. They had to be sharp and quick-witted, able to recognize patterns of both predators and prey, with impeccable memories and attention spans. Otherwise, we probably wouldn't have made it this far as a species.

Today's research has shown that when we feel hungry (when our blood glucose is low), the levels of norepinephrine in our body increases. Additionally, since our cells can no longer pull from our blood glucose for energy, they turn to our fat stores—our ketones—instead. This is a process known as "nutritional ketosis." Some research suggests that our brain actually functions more efficiently when fueled with ketones as opposed to glucose.

That is one of the elements behind the keto diet that appeals to so many people; if you eliminate sugars and carbohydrates (which your body turns into glucose, anyway) and drastically increase your healthy fat intake, all the fuel in your brain is coming from fat. This process is where "Fat to Fuel," the popular promotional phrase for the ketogenic diet, gets its origins.

While ketosis allows for better brain function that glucose, norepinephrine is drastically helpful in enhancing mental focus and memory storage. This hormone is closely related to adrenaline, also going by the name noradrenaline. While the two are chemically different and are used by different parts of the body, their similarity is in their function. They're both vital to our "fight or flight" response, kicking our blood pressure up a notch (or several) when we face extreme danger, excitement, or stress. Consequentially, in the face of hunger (a stressor), there's an uptick in norepinephrine to help our minds handle the situation.

One more perk that fasting can induce on our mental acuity: fasting, or going without food, triggers our sympathetic nervous system. This is responsible for our fight or flight responses. Even though we may be completely safe, our bodies register the lack of food as "danger." Our sympathetic nervous system revs up, sharpening our focus in an effort to help us "find food." It also triggers the release of human growth hormones and adrenaline, benefiting our bodies as well as our minds. Rigorous workouts while fasting have shown an exponential increase in fat loss and muscle gain, thanks to these specific hormones working together because they think we're "in danger."

How Fasting Burns Fat

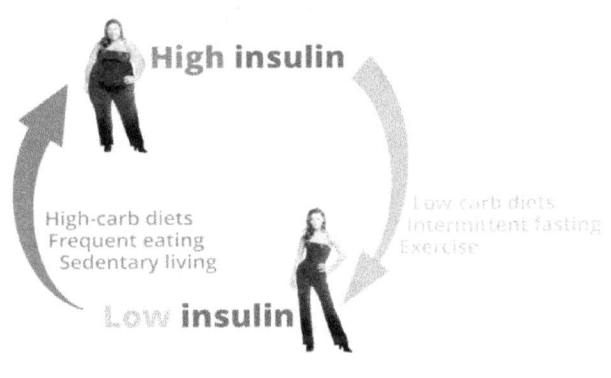

Adrenaline, norepinephrine, sympathetic nervous system, and hormone-sensitive lipase —in terms of fat breakdown during a fast, these are the key players. A lot of resources about intermittent fasting that can be found online give a vague description of the diet's fat burning capabilities at best—but they aren't hard to understand once you get around the biologic jargon. Every element of fasting's fat burning comes from hormones and processes that our body utilizes every day.

As mentioned in the last section, fasting can trigger our fight or flight response in a major way. This does more than just sharpen our mental abilities and enhance workout results. When our adrenaline and norepinephrine levels are high, our body's ability to burn fat is optimized. Our sympathetic nervous system keeps these two hormones high while we're fasting because technically, we're "starving" and our body is trying to help us find food.

Hormone-sensitive lipase triggers what is known as lipolysis, and also mobilizes our fat cells. Lipolysis is the process that our body uses to break down and utilize stored fatty acids and works similarly to how autophagy utilizes defective cells. Lipolysis is essential for processing triglycerides. On their own, triglycerides are relatively useless; however, hormone-sensitive lipase helps our bodies break them down into parts: 3 fatty acids (tri) and a molecule of glycerol (glyceride). Without it, foods that are high in triglycerides have nowhere to go except straight into our fat stores, resulting in weight gain. Just like how autophagy breaks down damaged cells into amino and fatty acids, lipolysis breaks down fats and turns them in to fuel.

Everything Runs on Hormones

In a video interview with Dr. Jason Fung, a popular name in the fasting and health community, he provided interesting insight into the role of calories in the human body. His claim: there isn't one. Calorie intake has literally no bearing on weight gain or weight loss; it all comes down to macronutrients and hormones.

For people who have gone their whole lives being told that eating less calories will help you lose weight, more calories will make you fat, you have to consume calories X times a day, and so on, this might be an uncomfortable concept. But from the perspective of our biology, it's an easy idea to grasp. Calories are determined by burning food and recording how much energy it gives off—but anything can have calories.

Vegetables, meats, cardboard, rocks... if it gives off energy when burned in a lab, it has calories. Obviously though, that doesn't mean that a strict diet of low-calorie sawdust is going to aid your weight loss, and by contrast, eating "a lot" of calories won't necessarily make you fat. That all depends on when and what you eat.

Gaining weight in fat is not caused directly by calories, which are more of a scientific construct and guideline than an actual biologic factor. Rather, our weight is affected by the hormones that certain foods produce or affect. Eating a spoonful of olive oil won't show much impact on our internal processes. However, eating the caloric equivalent in sugar will send your blood sugar through the roof, spiking your insulin levels, and leading to a domino effect of potential issues.

We begin facing issues with weight gain when we eat too many sugars or carbs, too often.

Every time you eat, your body processes some of that energy immediately and then puts the rest away to be used later. This goes into your liver and fat cells to be processed and stored. As Dr. Fung put in, "that's why we don't die in our sleep every night." While you sleep, you're in a natural state of fasting. This forces your body to tap into your stored energy to keep you going.

However, if you eat again (and again, and again...) before your body has a chance to use the energy that you're putting into storage, you'll only be stockpiling more and more into your fat stores. Eating many small meals a day or snacking throughout the day is not your friend when it comes to losing fat. It's very important to give your body a chance to utilize all the energy you're giving it, as we'll explore in the following chapter.

The important takeaway from Dr. Jason Fung's insight in terms of intermittent fasting is that even though you may feel a sense of discomfort or danger when your blood sugar is low, this is just your hormones reacting to the absence of something they're used to having: excess. As you continue with fasting intermittently, however, your hormones will be allowed to adjust and properly utilize the fat stores in your body. You'll quickly discover that it isn't the quantity or frequency of your eating schedule that affects your weight loss journey; it's the quality, and how your meals interact with your hormones.

Chapter 2:

Hormones vs Fasting, & How They Work Together

When starting any diet or new eating regimen, doctors and healthcare experts will advise you to keep tabs on your mood and energy levels. This is because the food you eat affects a lot more than just your muscles and fat; you'll also see significant changes in certain hormones. Everything in your body is very intricately connected, so it's important to know how it works together. If you're full of manic energy or constantly experiencing irregular heartbeats, it's probably time to stop your diet and reevaluate with your doctor. That said, dieting and caloric restriction can have some very positive, long-term effects on your vital hormones, as long as you implement them correctly.

Among a few others, insulin is a massive focal point here. Before starting an intermittent fast, having a solid understanding of insulin's role in your body is absolutely vital. It came up briefly in the previous chapter, but now it's getting a chance in the spotlight. If you already have a comprehensive understanding of insulin and the role it occupies in your body, the next few paragraphs might be old news.

Try strictly reading on from the perspective of how insulin affects you and your fast, rather than skimming ahead to the "new stuff."

Remember, a major player in successful weight loss is viewing how you eat (and the functions that accompany eating) in the light of your prospective weight loss plan. Knowing, as they say, is half the battle.

Insulin's Role in Your Body

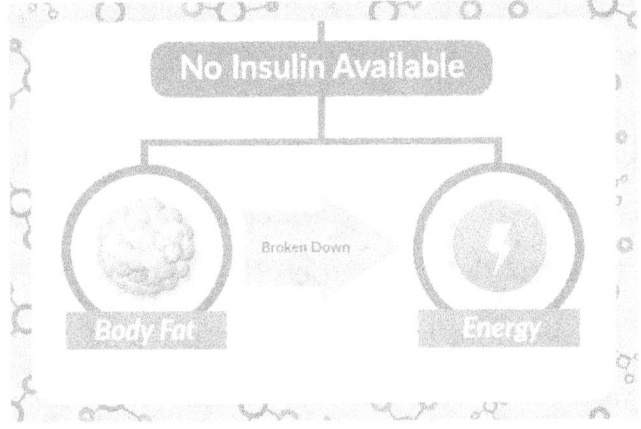

Without insulin, your body would all but cease to function. Imagine having excruciatingly low blood sugar (or blood glucose) at all times, with chronically malfunctioning metabolism and muscles, and you'll get an idea of what being devoid of insulin would do to your body. These issues are why patients with type 1 diabetes need supplementary insulin to survive.

If there isn't enough insulin in your body, your cells will begin to starve. Since there is no way for them to absorb the potential energy from glucose without insulin, they'll start searching for other means of energy. This search usually begins with the breakdown of your fat cells—not a good thing, in this situation. When your cells break down fat in this way, it releases excessive acids called ketones into your bloodstream, which can be life-threatening. The sudden influx of acid in your bloodstream can throw your whole system out of whack. This is known as ketoacidosis.

For most people, insulin is produced by the pancreas, a small organ located between the stomach and spine. (Those with type 1 diabetes are the exception, as their pancreas has failed to produce insulin.) Your pancreas is responsible for that boost of energy that accompanies a good meal. When you eat, it releases insulin into your bloodstream, which helps make metabolism possible. Insulin is also responsible for converting glucose (sugar) into energy and distribute it throughout your cells.

In addition to that immediate rush of energy you get from glucose conversion, insulin also aids your liver, fat cells, and muscles in storing the glucose you don't need right away. That stored glucose is released as you need it between meals, to help you feel satiated and energized longer. This also prevents your liver from over-producing glucose and helps to maintain healthy blood sugar levels. In order to stop your blood glucose from getting too high or too low, your insulin works with your organs and pancreas to keep your glucose levels between 70 and 110 mg/dl (with mg/dl denoting milligrams of glucose per 100 milliliters of blood.)

Keeping your blood sugar at a reasonably regulated level while you're going about your day is vital. If your blood glucose starts to get too low, you may begin to feel shaky, irritable, and/or fatigued. (Think of "low blood glucose" as the scientific name for "hangry.") If your blood glucose falls below 70 mg/dl this results in hypoglycemia. Hypoglycemia (the technical term for "really low blood glucose") can progress into confusion, irregular heartbeat, and even loss of consciousness. Luckily, your body has pretty strong indicators before that point to let you know it is time to get another boost.

Having abnormally high blood glucose isn't a good situation, either. Symptoms, in this case, include constantly feeling thirsty and excessive urination. High blood glucose can be a sign that you ate too much or too fast or haven't been getting enough exercise in general. The onset of this is usually much slower than the symptoms of low blood glucose, but both can have severe effects on your body and mind.

A common cause of both high blood glucose and weight gain is when your body over-produces insulin. This usually occurs when you eat highly processed foods or foods that are packed with carbs and sugars. When you eat things of this caliber, it's highly possible that your pancreas will drastically overestimate how much insulin it needs to produce. By the time you've rapidly burned through the amount of blood glucose you just consumed, there will still be an excess of insulin remaining with nothing left to do but cause problems. It can result in you feeling hungry much more quickly than you would otherwise, even if you don't need more food.

If the high levels of insulin in your blood successful trick you into eating more, your pancreas ends up producing more insulin to keep up, leading to a vicious cycle of hunger and potential weight gain. It can also overwork your pancreas, which can lead to a serious issue known as insulin resistance over time.

Insulin Resistance & Intermittent Fasting

Ideally, your cells will begin accepting glucose as energy as soon your pancreas sends insulin their way. Sometimes though, it takes a few more waves of insulin before your cells open up to accept the glucose—and this can be dangerous, depending on how long it takes. There's only so much insulin production your pancreas can keep up within a certain time frame. This is a common issue known as insulin resistance. It can have severe effects including insulin deficiency or pre-diabetes, both of which have some wild effects on your body's fat storage and blood sugar.

Weight gain usually accompanies insulin resistance, because your cells aren't taking as much glucose out of your bloodstream as they should be, there's a lot of excesses to deal with. After your body detects that glucose has been in your blood for a while, it assumes it is "unnecessary" and stores it for later. But it is necessary—just inaccessible. As you eat more in an effort to feel energized, your body is "helpfully" putting a lot of that blood glucose directly into your fat cells. Consequentially, above-average waistlines and extra stomach fat are common in folks with insulin resistance. And in almost every case, insulin resistance accompanies obesity.

While weight goes up due to excessive eating, energy goes down. This isn't the most dangerous symptom of insulin resistance, but it is more noticeable in day-to-day life. Since insulin resistance restricts the blood glucose that reaches your cells, there is significantly less of your body's main fuel source being utilized, and a lot of it being mistakenly stored as fat, which tends to slow us down after a while.

This is a highly nuanced condition, so although the long-term effects can be severe, it often goes unnoticed and unchecked. The symptoms are not necessarily unique (including sugar cravings, fatigue, acne, excess stomach fat, etc.), so naturally, not a lot of people go seeking medical advice when they arise. The main causes of insulin resistance are equally inconspicuous: rapid weight gain, insufficient exercise, eating a high-carb diet, and loss of sleep. Due to the general normality of the causes and symptoms, many people with insulin resistance go on to fully develop type 2 diabetes as a result of the untreated disorder.

This is where intermittent fasting comes in to play.

In recent years, fasting has been explored as a potential cure for type 2 diabetes and has shown considerable potential in the reversal of insulin resistance. Even if you don't have insulin resistance, it is a beneficial diet for improving your insulin's function. If you do have insulin resistance (even if you don't know it yet), intermittent fasting can be the step needed to figure it out and nip it in the bud.

During the periods that you are not eating during your intermittent fast—usually between 12 and 20 hours, which the next chapter will discuss further—there are some significant changes in your blood glucose and insulin levels.

During this "fasted" state, your insulin and glucose levels are both low (between 70 and 100 mg/dl), giving your pancreas and cells a much-needed break. When your body stops burning the glucose obtained in your "fed" state, it turns to the place where your insulin stored the extra glucose for later use: your fat cells.

Your body does not burn fat while you are in the "fed" state. If you are fed, you are not burning fat. To state it directly makes it seem obvious, but it isn't usually the first thought to come to mind when our stomachs are growling. In intermittent fasting, the "fed" state is usually the 4–8-hour window where you may eat whatever you like. During this time, instead of going for your fat reserves, your body is using the immediately obtained glucose as fuel—which is totally fine. However, think about it in terms of a regular eating schedule (not intermittent fasting or dieting). Usually, people have 3 meals a day, with snacks and drinks in between, and really only "fast" when they're asleep. This keeps us energized and quiets our stomachs, sure—but as soon as we eat and insulin is released, the fat burning process comes to a screeching halt. In this context, "healthy snacks" do not equate to losing weight.

The regular eating pattern that so many people fall into during their busy day-to-day lives is a nasty conduit for insulin resistance. Studies have shown that even the slightest caloric intake, such as putting creamer in your coffee, stops fat loss and autophagy in their tracks. Stop the process too often, and you'll start to build up an immunity to it happening at all. Intermittent fasting's unique and adaptable guidelines have shown phenomenal results on reversing insulin resistance and weight loss because during the hours where you are not eating a thing, your body has nothing to burn but fat.

In addition to your levels of blood glucose and insulin dropping (and staying down) during your fasting hours, there is also an increase in your growth hormone and norepinephrine (the hormone released in your blood that affects mood and increases heart rate.) Both of these hormones "work against" insulin, in the sense that they complete the opposite functions. Insulin works to distribute and store blood glucose; growth hormones and norepinephrine burn it up. Just think about how hungry you were all the time during your childhood growth-spurts. This combination of hormonal adjustments along with the general caloric reduction that naturally happens with intermittent fasting is a powerful method for burning off excess fat. Norepinephrine is especially important to this function: as it increases (and raises your blood pressure) your metabolism picks up speed. You begin burning more calories than you take in. This is absolutely vital to healthy weight loss, and by proxy, the reversal and prevention of insulin resistance.

Insulin vs. Autophagy

Since autophagy was such a key focal point in the last chapter, it is definitely worth mentioning that insulin and autophagy do not get along. When your insulin and blood glucose spike, even just a little, autophagy completely stops. So unfortunately, snacking and autophagy don't mix. It does make sense though: by eating whenever you feel hungry (that is, whenever your blood glucose is low), you're eliminating the healthy stressor that accompanies a dip in insulin and blood glucose. Autophagy is a powerful biologic function that allows us to adapt and our bodies and immune systems to become stronger, but if there is never any mild discomfort to trigger it, what would be the point in furthering the process?

From autophagy's perspective, it would look like we had reached the peak of our necessary evolution.

Leptin, Glucagon, & Ghrelin: Meet Your Hunger Hormones

You might not know their names, but beyond a shadow of a doubt, you have become very well acquainted with these hormones throughout your life. Leptin is the hormone that tells your brain when you're full, and ghrelin tells you (loudly) when you're hungry. Glucagon is produced in the pancreas like insulin, but it affects your liver. All these hormones work very closely with each other and with insulin, and they're all peptide hormones, so their distribution and functions are all linked together. Understanding each of these hormones individually can greatly improve the quality of your fast because you'll know what your body is really trying to tell you. It is a lot easier to "listen to your body" once you're speaking the same language.

Peptide hormones are hormones that can travel freely through your bloodstream without assistance. This differs for other hormones like cortisol or adrenaline, which may need a carrier protein to travel through your blood. In general, peptide hormones oversee the regulation of your automatic biologic functions, as well as energy and nutrients storage. They are released into your system as prohormones, meaning they are inactive precursors to those hormones until affected by an external process. Then, once they're activated, peptide hormones can trigger immediate (but short-lived) bodily functions, like the conversion of blood glucose to energy via insulin.

When your blood glucose drops and there is no more glucose left for your cells to absorb, glucagon kicks in to help convert the glycogen previously stored in your liver into glucose.

This is part of how you can burn fat and maintain energy while fasting. Once your other hormonal reactions trigger the release of glucagon, you know you're on the right track. After the glucose converted from your liver is absorbed and used up, then your cells turn to your fat stores for an energy source (as long as you don't raise your blood glucose again for a while.)

Ghrelin is mainly responsible for triggering hunger. It's produced in our stomach and works by travelling through our bloodstream to our brains and telling us to seek out food. Once ghrelin becomes accustomed to your daily eating habits, it will start sending signals to your brain accordingly. This is why you generally feel hungry around the same times each day, regardless of how much you had in your previous meal. This aspect of ghrelin can make the beginning of an intermittent fast a bit miserable. Since you'll be modifying your eating habits so dramatically, your ghrelin levels might be equally dramatic, signaling to your brain that you might be dying because you missed breakfast. This will only last a few days though because like all of our hormones and biologic processes, ghrelin is very adaptable. Once you've been on an intermittent fast for about a week, ghrelin will have had a chance to learn your new routine.

Fun fact: ghrelin also has an effect on your taste receptors. If you've ever eaten something while ravenously hungry and it tasted better than anything you've ever had—even if it was just a bag of chips—you can thank ghrelin for that. Amplified hunger can lead to amplified taste.

Leptin works directly with your body's fat cells and your brain's hypothalamus. Its primary role is to help us maintain body weight, and control long-term energy expenditure and distribution. For the most part, leptin is a satiation hormone—the opposite of ghrelin. It helps us feel full longer by inhibiting other hunger hormones from moving too quickly to our brains. Leptin, however, also plays a major part obesity and issues losing weight.

Since it's connected to our fat cells, the amount of leptin produced by our bodies will increase if we add body fat and decrease if we lose it. If you rapidly lose a lot of body fat, there will suddenly be a lot less leptin going to your brain, leading to a disproportionate amount of ghrelin. This can send your hunger through the roof, making it extremely hard to resist food cravings, and giving you some of the worse symptoms of hypoglycemia.

In that regard, another reason that you'll feel so famished for the first few days of your fast is because by losing body weight, you're decreasing leptin but having no effect on ghrelin, so more ghrelin is able to tell your brain "Hey, please eat food right now." After a week or so, these hormones should balance back out, as ghrelin adapts to your new eating routine, and leptin stabilizes.

Fasting in Men vs. Women—What's the Difference?

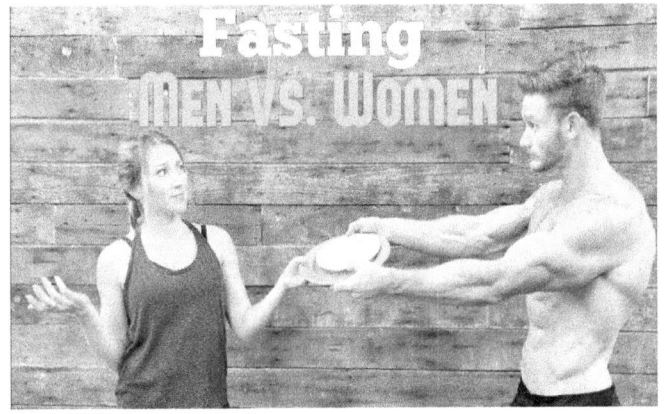

Across the Internet and dietary guides, there are quite a few sources and articles that grossly overemphasize the potential dangers for women when it comes to fasting. Some of the arguments that get thrown around are that it can decrease thyroid activity, drastically mess up hormones, and damage to the reproductive system. And while these points have a general semblance of scientific backing, they are not entirely accurate and can be easily mitigated if handled correctly.

Technically, it is true that "fasting slows your thyroid." Your thyroid is functioning slower when you are in the fasted state. However, your thyroid is also slower between regular meals. While intermittent fasting can slow it down for long, you probably aren't doing any permanent damage. An easy way to tell if your thyroid has, in fact, slowed down in a more permanent way is if you start feeling extremely cold all the time. Feeling cold while fasting is normal for everyone, men and women alike, but feeling chronically cold could be a sign of a slowing thyroid.

When discussing the hormonal impacts of fasting, there is quite a bit of biology-related jargon to unpack. Men and women both experience around the same level of hormonal changes while practicing intermittent fasting. However, women are typically more sensitive (chemically) to changes in hunger-related hormones, including leptin, ghrelin, and insulin. When changes occur that drastically increase the level of hunger hormones being produced, women are more likely to have severe reactions. This is thanks to a protein-like substance known as kisspeptin.

Men and women both produce kisspeptin, but women produce more of it. Kisspeptin is your body's precursor to GnRH—a hormone secreted from your brain that directly controls ovulation and reproductive hormones in both men and women. In order to help your body conserve energy and promote healthy reproduction, kisspeptin is extremely sensitive to our hunger hormones. So, naturally, the fact the women automatically produce more kisspeptin explains their general increased reactions to hunger.

What is known as your gonadotropin-releasing hormone, or GnRH, is secreted from your brain's hypothalamus, which controls your autonomic nervous system and sends signals to the pituitary gland. GnRH works directly with the reproductive mechanisms and hormones of both men and women, stimulating the production of testosterone in men and progesterone and estrogen in women. It is also responsible for triggering the release of two hormones that control nearly every pubertal and reproductive process of our bodies: follicle-stimulating hormone (FSH) and luteinizing hormones (LH).

FSH is the hormone that induces the development and growth of our body's pubertal and reproductive processes. Similarly, LH is responsible for stimulating ovulation in females and the release of androgen in males. Since both of these processes are directly affected by kisspeptin, it makes sense that our reproductive and hormonal processes are linked so closely with our hunger hormones.

This is a great survival mechanism, especially in females. Since the female reproductive system usually utilizes an increased amount of energy to create eggs, ovulation might get out of whack at the start of your fast. If your body thinks you're starving, it isn't going to want to try and reproduce because you need that energy. Unfortunately, it's also the catalyst for making fasting a more uncomfortable endeavor for women. With that being said, there is nothing stating that women can't fast, regardless of what concerned friends and half-accurate articles might tell you. It might just take a bit more mental resilience from the get-go, and some additional strategizing. You'll read more about this in the next chapter.

Chapter 3:

Intermittent Fasting in Daily Life

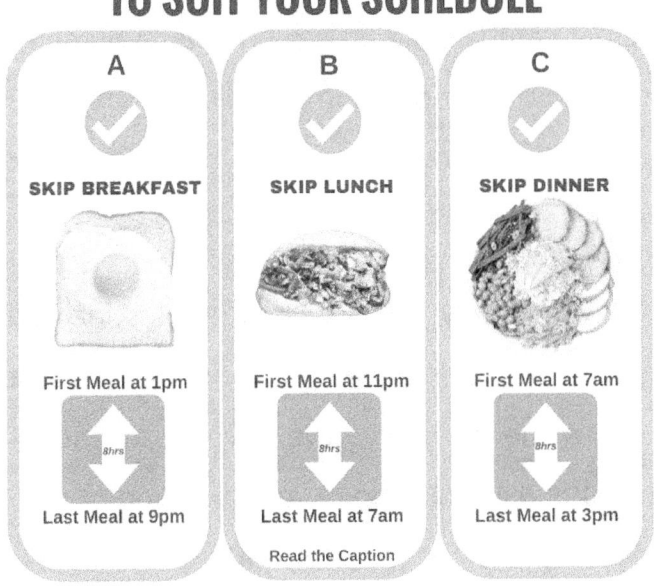

INTERMITTENT FASTING
TO SUIT YOUR SCHEDULE

A	B	C
SKIP BREAKFAST	SKIP LUNCH	SKIP DINNER
First Meal at 1pm	First Meal at 11pm	First Meal at 7am
8hrs	8hrs	8hrs
Last Meal at 9pm	Last Meal at 7am	Last Meal at 3pm
	Read the Caption	

As you've read, intermittent fasting isn't like many other diet plans. It has not only own unique health benefits, but also a unique set of warnings and necessary lifestyle adjustments. Unlike other diets that require you to watch what you eat but not when you might not be able to just right into intermittent fasting while keeping your social and personal life unchanged. Changing what you eat can be easy; changing when you eat— or for some people, completely relearning all your eating habits—can have much more of an impact on daily life.

This isn't to say that intermittent fasting will have negative impacts on your life. It's just going to be new. If you've never fasted long-term before, your body and hormones may require a longer adjustment period before you feel "normal" again. And while going into an intermittent fast doesn't need as much actual "meal planning" as other diets, as you'll read in the next chapter, it does require more premeditation, research, and possibly day-by-day planning.

Making the Transition

Although everyone's experience with intermittent fasting is unique, there is one massively common warning that most practitioners share. The first few days (3–5, by most accounts) are going to be the worst. Luckily, though, our bodies are made to adapt to new situations—even if our brains take a little extra convincing. Here are some helpful tips to help your mind, body, and hormones adapt to your new routine.

Cut the Snacks

One of the most helpful strategies when considering trying an intermittent fast is to stop snacking. That's it. You can still eat 3 meals a day at whatever times you usually would; just don't have a snack in between meals. If food cravings start creeping up on you, try drinking the calorie-free beverages that are allowed during your fast, like black coffee or unsweetened tea. Then, if you're starting your fast on a 16/8 regimen, all you'll have to do is eliminate either breakfast or dinner from your daily routine. Worry about cutting out the small things first and work your way up from there; your body will thank you.

Eliminating snacks from your daily routine for at least a few days prior to your fast will be incredibly helpful for building your fasting strategy. For some of us, grabbing a power bar or snagging samples from grocery store vendors isn't something we think very hard about. But if you make the conscious effort not to have any calories between your regular meals, you'll be lowering your general insulin levels, curbing your cravings, and training your mind to go for a mug of tea when your stomach is growling, rather than a sugar-and-carb loaded treat.

This method will also help you gauge your personal nutritional needs and can be a good time to start experimenting with adding more nutrient-dense foods to your meals, such as dark greens and other vegetables. Without sporadic snacks to affect your insulin and glucose levels, you'll be able to get a much more accurate feel for which foods and meal plans keep you feeling satiated and energized the longest. In this regard, everyone's body is different. We all have our own unique nutritional needs based on general health and lifestyles, so there isn't a "standard" to set you up with as you go into your fast.

This may also be a good time to start exploring specific diets to combine intermittent fasting with: if a proper amount of foods with high-fat contents make you feel amazing, maybe you would benefit from a more ketogenic diet while you fast. And if those leafy greens are more satisfying than you'd previously imagined, you could look into how a vegetarian or vegan plan could optimize the fasting benefits. You'll get a glimpse of how intermittent fasting works with these diets and others in the next chapter.

Don't Let Hunger Turn to Binging

Once you've cut out snacks and then breakfast or dinner, your intermittent fast will have officially begun. Although a transition period of a few days will be beneficial, your body is still going to be a little baffled when you start fasting for real on a regular basis. During the first week, you might be amazed at how hungry you are before your scheduled eating window. This is normal, but don't let your body fool you into gorging down excessive food once the time comes.

In the elongated company of hunger, you might find yourself spending more and more time fantasizing about all the foods you are going to eat when the clock strikes Meal Time. And you might want to eat a whole lot at once. These are your cravings talking. While it is important to listen to your body, it is also important to recognize that sometimes your body is incorrect, and you are only craving a burger and fries because you just saw that ad on TV, not because you need them to survive. Sip your coffee or tea—or better yet, a glass of water—and turn your attention to something else for the time being.

Once it is time for food, start off with something jam-packed with nutrients, healthy fats, potassium, and the like. A serving of mixed nuts or a hearty side of vegetables is great places to start. It is also beneficial to eat at a moderate pace, but it's understandable if you accidentally inhale breakfast for the first few days—as long as you are not eating an excessive amount of "junk foods." Once you have had a healthy dose of vitamins and fats, your body should stop feeling ravenously hungry. At that point, it is probably a lot safer to pull out a bag of chips.

The main issue with scarfing down your first meal is that your blood glucose levels will go from zero to a hundred (metaphorically speaking) very quickly. This can lead to feeling hungry a lot sooner and crashing harder between meals in your eating window. It is better if you can pace yourself, letting your pancreas and leptin process how much you are eating as you eat it, instead of scrambling to catch up after the fact. This way it will be easier to tell when you are actually full, and you won't blow your insulin levels out of proportion.

Avoid Empty Calories

When thinking about what foods you'll have during your eating window, junk foods and heavily refined carbohydrates should be an afterthought. Dessert is fine in moderation, but if you're having pastries for your main course, that will deprive your body of the vital nutrients it needs to keep going strong. Yes, you can eat whatever fits your regular diet during the eating window—but it's important to remember that you'll be consuming less food in the day on average, so healthy and nutrient-rich foods should fill most of your plate.

Light portions of healthy fats are an excellent alternative to full meals of processed carbohydrates. You need less of them, which makes time and room for eating other nutritious foods. Fats also stick with you much better, making you feel satiated for longer into your fasting period.

Persevere

While this one seems obvious prior to beginning your fast, you may reach a point in the first week or so where you'll need to be reminded of it. A huge mistake that many new fasters make is giving up too soon, due to the initial negative side effects. If you truly want to see the positive effects of the fast over time, it's important to push through the rough transition period.

This may be easier said than done, but there are many ways to make fasting a more comfortable and beneficial experience, even during the rough patches. Your environment can be a major factor. If you're constantly going out with friends or going over to family gatherings outside of your eating window, this can make fasting seem a lot more like pulling teeth. Try going out more during your eating window, and using your fasting period to exercise, focus on your work or chores, or rest. Invite friends and family to hang out in your personal environment, so you have more control over the food cravings you might be exposed to in the first week.

Although it is important to push through the first week of fasting to achieve the pinnacle benefits, there is no shame in stopping after that point.

Many people who have experimented with intermittent fasting stopped after 10–14 days and still saw some impressive weight loss benefits. If fasting is still making you feel irritable or exhausted after a trial run, maybe it just isn't for you. There are plenty of other diet plans out there, but at least you'll be able to say that you gave intermittent fasting a strong shot.

<u>Don't Forget to Drink Water</u>

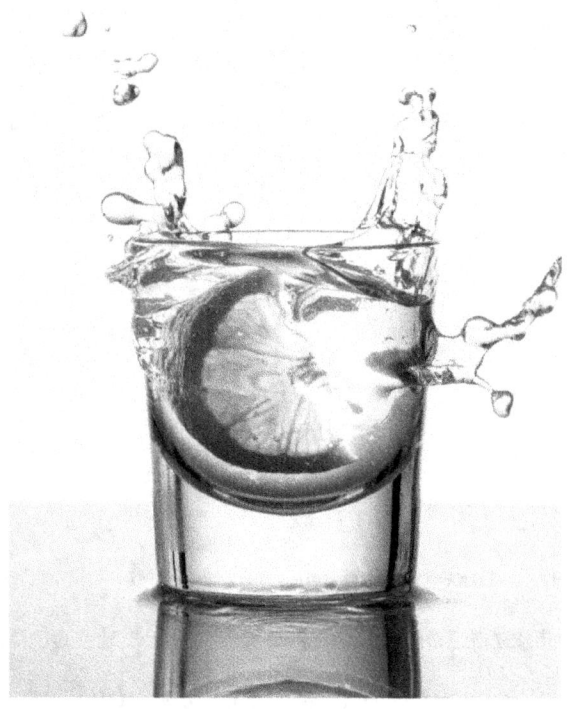

More often than not, even when we aren't fasting, hunger pangs are a sign that we're thirsty or dehydrated. Our stomach is telling us that it wants something to go in, but not what. And usually, a glass of water can be enough to satiate us until the next meal. But since hunger pangs are the same whether we need liquid or solids, many of us resort to food to tide us over. This can lead to inadvertently overeating and, in some cases, dehydration.

While it's always important to stay hydrated, increasing your water intake while fasting is vital. It can be amazingly beneficial to add electrolyte to the water bottle you use regularly, in order to get the combination of hydration and energy maintenance. We'll cover which electrolytes are the most important and why in

Popular Timeframes for Intermittent Fasting

A few names you may have heard intermittent fasting referred to include "alternate day fasting" and the "Eat-Stop-Eat" method. All of these are acceptable ways to practice intermittent fasting, and each has their own unique appeals. Unlike completely fasting, you are certainly allowed to eat during any intermittent fasting plan; however, there are long timeframes between your "feeding hours."

Eat-Stop-Eat: 16/8

16/8 Fasting Protocol Over 24 Hours

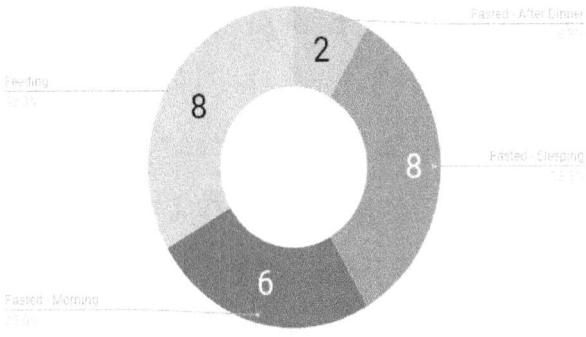

One of the most popular takes on intermittent fasting is the 16/8 method. "16/8" is a breakdown of the hours in the day, and how to spend them: 16 hours fasting, with an 8-hour eating window.

This is a commonly recommended plan for beginners since it isn't too much of a stretch from how you're probably used to eating. 16 hours of not eating may seem like a daunting number to look at but consider the fact that when we sleep, our bodies are naturally in a "fasted" state. That's typically about 6–8 hours that you won't even be awake for. When the day rolls around, that leaves only 10–8 hours for you to deal with.

The 16/8 method is very flexible, and it is likely that no intermittent fasters implement it exactly the same. The 8-hour feeding window does not mean that you'll be eating continuously for 8 hours (even if you feel like it for the first few days of your fast). All it means is that you only have those 8 consecutive hours to be in a "fed" state. You can eat, snack, and drink beverages just like you would on a normal diet. But once that 8 hours is up, all caloric intake stops for the next 16 hours.

Even without being on a diet, you can probably recognize a pattern in what times of the day you eat. "Breakfast, lunch, and dinner" times vary from person to person, as in, they are not a permanent aspect of our biology. The breakdown is pretty simple: we eat when we're hungry and when our blood glucose is low, but as we fall into the patterns of our daily lives, our hormones start to catch on... and try to help us out. No matter how much you eat for breakfast, you'll probably feel your stomach growling around the time you usually eat lunch. However, this doesn't mean you need food right then; it just means you've inadvertently set a biologic alarm clock for yourself. If you skip lunch, your hunger will subside after a while, and you likely won't feel hungry again until your usual dinner time.

While how you plan when you eat is entirely dependent on your preferences and your daily schedule, one thing to make sure of is that you are eating during the same time each day. This is most vital for your own comfort, and it will make the transition to intermittent fasting much easier. Intermittent fasting works with that concept of our "internal alarm clock."

Many people on the regime have said that it only took them a few days of strictly following the 16/8 plan for their bodies to catch on.

After four or five days, most people claim that they no longer feel hunger pains 3 times a day

—just around the time that they ate the previous day.

If you typically have busy early mornings and slow, mellow evenings, you might want to try an eating window from 6AM–2PM and spend the rest of the day fasting. In this situation, the only meal you're "missing" would be dinner. However, the stigma of breakfast being the most important meal of the day is almost entirely a myth, as we can gather from fasting's ability to enhance our cognitive function. Don't let that concept exclusively influence your planning process. If you'd rather be fasting during the busier parts of your day, or if you often have dinner plans with family and friends, you could try an eating window from 4PM–12AM. If part of the window overlaps your usual bedtime that's perfectly fine, as long as you don't start eating outside of it. Sleeping off a few hours of your potential feeding time only means that your fast the next day will be a bit longer, and assuming you eat again at the usual time, your hunger shouldn't see much difference.

Advanced Take on 16/8

If the 16/8 method is too much of a breeze for you, or if you want to see more of the fast's benefits, you can cut down on your eating hours and add to those you spend fasting. Some popular windows are 18/6 and 20/4 (also known as the "Warrior diet"). Especially with the 20/4 plan you'll only be able to squeeze in one meal a day with a snack or two, but you'll see a massive increase in benefits such as autophagy and fat breakdown.

After around 16 hours of fasting is when most experts believe the positive effects start to accumulate exponentially, so if you get comfortable with intermittent fasting and want a challenge, the results will be well worth it.

Alternate Day Fasting

Alternate day fasting (ADF)

| Feed day | Fast day |
| Day of ad libitum feeding | Day of 75% restriction |

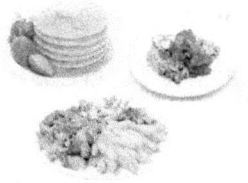 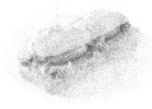

Alternate day fasting is another commonly used approach to intermittent fasting. As the helpfully literal name suggests, in this method, you fast every other day. On the days in between fasting, you may eat however and whatever you like, within your own restrictions. Instead of restricting your eating to the 16/8 method, you are allowed 24 hours of unobstructed eating, and then fast for the next 24 hours.

One difference in this approach is that, in some cases, practitioners might consume up to 500 calories on their "fasting" day.

Alternate day fasting has shown more inconsistencies in hunger levels than the eat-stop-eat method, but the common agreement is that this 500-calorie allowance makes the rest of the 24 hours much more bearable. Do take note, however, that these 500 calories should be consumed around the same time—not throughout the day. In the fasting state, if your blood glucose increases even slightly, many of the processes occurring in your cells will come to a sudden stop. While having a light snack once per fasting day won't have much effect, spreading that out could negate the effects of the fast while also not making you feel any less hungry.

"Crescendo" Fasting for Women and Beginners

Crescendo fasting follows the same principals as 16/8 fasting. The difference, however, is that instead of implementing the 16/8 method every day, you start by following it for two or three nonconsecutive days a week. Typically, after two weeks you can increase the number of days you spend fasting, so long as you're comfortable and seeing the benefits so far.

This method that is one of the healthier ways for women, especially, to commit to the start of an intermittent fast. It's also a good idea in general for anyone who is unsure if it's the right choice or anyone who has health concerns that may make a fully committing to an intermittent fast risky. By only fasting for a couple days out of the week, you can get a feel for how your hormones and energy will be affected during the process, and you will still see an increase in autophagy compared to usual eating habits. But the immediate negative effects on those with higher fasting risks (women and people with insomnia or high stress) won't be nearly as severe as they would be by jumping straight into a full fast.

By easing your body into fasting intermittently, you can greatly extend the adjustment period for your body. If you decide you enjoy the benefits of fasting and want to attempt it every day, or six days a week, it won't be a major shock to your body and hormones like jumping straight in might be. For people who have increased stressors in their lives, this method can help mitigate the bodily stress that fasting adds. And for women, easing your body into fasting can help with reproductive health and regular ovulation over the course of the rest of your fast.

During the days that you are not fasting during this plan, doing strenuous workout routines can be a great way to keep the energy you get from fasting in effect. On fasting days, yoga and light cardio will keep you moving without draining all your energy for the day. During both types of days, it is absolutely crucial to stay adequately hydrated. Increasing your fluid intake will help you stay active, and will also help to minimize food cravings, both on fasting days and non-fasting ones.

While this can be a great way to test the waters of fasting, it is still important to remember that your health is your primary concern. If during the two or three fasting days you feel incredibly sluggish, irritable, or have more trouble sleeping than usual, you should consult with your doctor before introducing more fasting days into your plan.

Fasting Period: Dos & Don'ts

When you are in your fasting state, whether it's for 20 hours or 12, you cannot consume any calories (Of course, this excludes the small 500-calorie allowance for alternate day fasting) .

Any caloric intake during this period will completely reset many of the active benefits that only occur when you're fasting, regardless of how long you've been fasting for. Autophagy will stop, and if you inadvertently spike your insulin or blood glucose, the fat breakdown will cease as well. And depending on what you eat, you may run the risk of feeling even more hungry after an accidental snack, further ruining the effects for that period.

This isn't to say nothing can enter your body when you're in the fasted state. It isn't a dry fast. You are more than welcome to consume any calorie-free drinks, such as tea and plain black coffee. It is also in your best interest to drink a lot of water. These can be hot or iced, but unfortunately, you cannot add sugar or sweeteners to them since these have calories and raise blood sugar. If you have a favorite coffee blend or tea selection that you can take without modifications, you may want to stock up on those before your fast.

Diet soda is also an option but at your own discretion. Some artificial sweeteners run the risk of slightly increasing your blood glucose, which can negate your fast. Stevia, in moderation, is the best option, since it doesn't interact with your insulin or glucose levels nearly as much as other artificial sweeteners. And diet soda is calorie free. Just keep an eye out for symptoms of increased hunger (a sign of insulin increase) if you choose to drink it.

Teas & Their Benefits

In general, tea is an ancient beverage that has been enjoyed across the decade for its health benefits, a variety of flavors, energy and mental enhancement, and ease of access. While you're on a fast, almost all this variety is still available to you. Unless teas have added fruit or sugar, they won't break your fast.

Green tea is absolutely incredible, regardless of whether or not you're fasting. Green tea alone is a powerful antioxidant and source of light caffeine. If you have a cup while you're fasting, it can give you a smooth caffeine rush and increase the benefits of autophagy, antioxidizing processes, and fat burning. When you aren't fasting, green tea can be a way to help fight inflammation and maintain healthy metabolic functions.

Black tea has some of the health benefits of green teas, but in terms of antioxidizing properties, it isn't quite as strong. However, if you aren't a coffee person but need a reliable source of caffeine to keep you sane, black tea packs more of a punch than green. It not only has more caffeine per cup, but it can also help you have a source of calmer, less jittery energy that won't have you crashing in a few hours.

You may need to be more careful with herbal teas. While there is significantly more variety among them, this also means that some manufacturers have gotten more creative with the ingredients they've added. You want to make sure your choice of herbal tea is strictly the herbs—no additives. Some herbal teas might have a more creative flavor profile by adding clumps of caramelized sugar, bits of dehydrated fruit, or artificial flavors. While these make for delicious drinks, they will break your fast. But as long as your herbal tea has no calories or sugar, have as much as you'd like. Peppermint, chamomile, lavender, and turmeric are just a few of the deliciously healthy herbal teas available.

Medications & Fasting

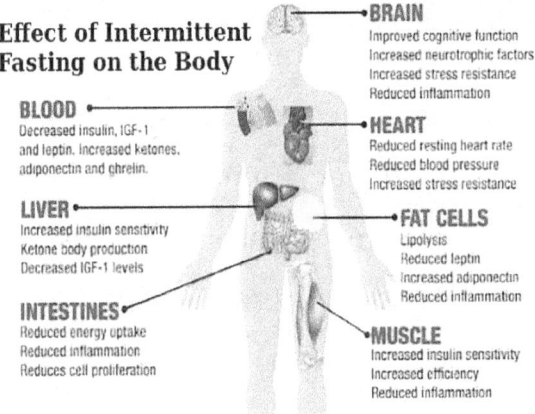

Effect of Intermittent Fasting on the Body

BRAIN
Improved cognitive function
Increased neurotrophic factors
Increased stress resistance
Reduced inflammation

BLOOD
Decreased insulin, IGF-1 and leptin. Increased ketones, adiponectin and ghrelin.

HEART
Reduced resting heart rate
Reduced blood pressure
Increased stress resistance

LIVER
Increased insulin sensitivity
Ketone body production
Decreased IGF-1 levels

FAT CELLS
Lipolysis
Reduced leptin
Increased adiponectin
Reduced inflammation

INTESTINES
Reduced energy uptake
Reduced inflammation
Reduces cell proliferation

MUSCLE
Increased insulin sensitivity
Increased efficiency
Reduced inflammation

If you take medications or vitamin supplements on daily basis, you are welcome to keep taking them as usual. However, you should check to see if they contain any carbs or calories before you take them during the fasting period. On a very technical level, even consuming one calorie could break your fast. Fish oil pills or gel capsules also have the potential to break your fast, because whatever oil they are suspended in (usually coconut or vegetable) can trigger a metabolic response. You are still welcome to take them—just wait until you're having your first meal of the day, so you don't ruin your fast.

Certain supplements even work well with your fast, which you'll explore in the next chapter. However, if you are on strong doses of prescription medication, you should consult your doctor before committing to a full intermittent fast. Some medications can cause severe damage or discomfort if taken on an empty stomach, or if you aren't eating regularly.

The Grey Areas

Since intermittent fasting is still being tested and researched today, there are some things that not all experts agree on. For example, there are some beverages that may or may not break your fast—depending on the expert you ask.

A commonly consumed drink (and an oddly controversial one while fasting) is simply a glass of water with a splash of lemon juice. Lemon juice has some wonderful effects on your cells and digestion, but consequentially, it might also trigger a metabolic response that could break your fast. Some experts argue that the downsides of consuming lemon juice during your fast pale in comparison to the benefits, but on a very technical level, you would still be consuming a calorie or two. If lemon water is a beverage you can't live without, inconclusive evidence means that at least it isn't the worst thing you could be drinking. Have a glass at your own discretion if you desire but stay in tune with your body and watch for any signs that your insulin levels have increased.

Powdered pre-workout drinks are another beverage that experts hotly debate. The general consensus for this one is that "not all pre-workouts are created equal." Before you have one during your fast, check the carbs. If it has any, that means it has dietary "fillers" or appetite suppressants, and it will break your fast.

But if it has no carbs or sugar, with the bulk of the nutrients in the protein and fats, you should be okay to consume it during your fasting period.

Alcohol vs. Fasting

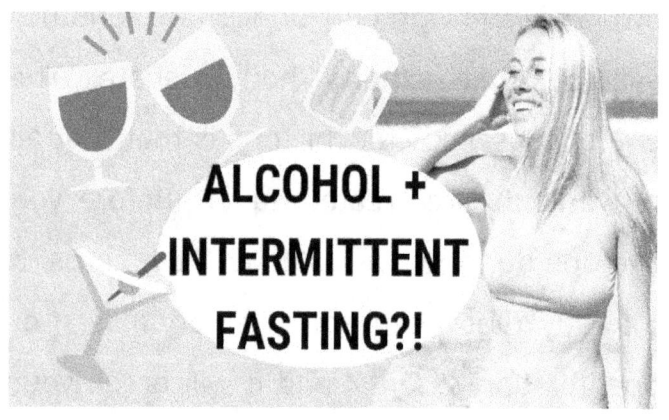

Unlike the other two drinks mentions, one thing is certain about alcohol: it will break your fast. Alcohol has about 7 calories per gram, which mean it triggers your metabolic processes and breaks you out of the fasting state. However, it is definitely not something you want to use on purpose to initially break your fast.

Since it is proven that alcohol breaks a fast, that isn't the factor that's in the grey area. The part of alcohol that not everybody agrees on is whether it should be consumed during a fast or not. Some people argue that as long as you aren't consuming it frequently, alcohol shouldn't be too detrimental to your diet. Others say that the cons of having alcohol on an intermittent fast out-weight the pros, and that it should just be avoided until your fast is over.

The way that alcohol is processed and metabolized is a complex process, involving your brain, liver, and many hormones and enzymes. When you have alcohol on a regular eating day or a full stomach, you'll notice that you don't feel the effects as quickly as you might on an empty stomach. Among other reasons, this is because your body already has food and nutrients that it's processing, and the alcohol is waiting for its turn. This can lead to overconsumption of alcohol in order to feel the effects sooner, which in turn causes everyone's favorite thing to wake up to the next morning.

Alcohol consumption while fasting is a whole different ball game. Even if you've eaten prior to having alcohol (which you should definitely do), your stomach and small intestines are still relatively empty. This leads to a few different domino effects—some negative, some positive.

Some people enjoy the fact that the alcohol is going to hit your system way faster than usual, which reduces the chance to have too much, and therefore reduces the chance of a hangover the next day. One or two pints of beer might get you as buzzed as a few shots of liquor would. Additionally, while you're fasting your body is in a sort of perpetual "detoxing" state, which contributes to less negative symptoms the day after having a few drinks.

All of that, however, also means that the alcohol you've consumed is also going to leave your body much quicker. Although this can help with the next day's hangover, that's where the positive effects of the expedited metabolism stop. Metabolizing alcohol this quickly actually poses some health risks if you aren't careful. Yes, it will hit you faster and you may not drink as much, but this also results in your liver and enzymes scrambling to keep up with the proper metabolic processes. Instead of alcohol being processed with or after the other things in your stomach, it hits you so fast that your enzymatic functions put everything else on hold to keep up.

One of the molecules produced when you metabolize alcohol is acetaldehyde, which is about 30 times as toxic as alcohol itself. On a typical day, this isn't usually an issue—but with how much fasting speeds up your alcohol metabolism, your body runs a real risk of not being able to keep up with processing and breaking down acetaldehyde, which can be serious to your health. So, while it's in your system, virtually all other processes come to a stop until it's gone.

In addition to this, alcohol also has some negative effects on our central nervous system.

This is pretty common knowledge—a major part of getting buzzed, tipsy, or drunk is the slowing of your central nervous system. However, on a fast, your central nervous system is seeing a lot of action between handling a new stressor, autophagy, and ketosis. If you have alcohol on a fast, be aware that it isn't going to have any positive effects in those regards. Many processes that intermittent fasting would usually induce, including fat burning, will completely stop until the alcohol is out of your system.

If you're going to have alcohol, there's nothing to stop you. There are certain timeframes that are better to have it than others. If you've committed to an alternate day or crescendo fast, pick a day when you are eating regularly to consume alcohol. If you're on a 16/8 fast or any variation thereof, you should definitely consume carbohydrates before alcohol. This will give your liver a buffet and soften the effects of acetaldehyde. Even if you're trying to maintain a primarily low-carb diet, consuming carbs before a drink will help you out a lot. 20–30 grams of carbs, maximum, should be enough to aid the process.

How to Properly Break Your Fast

"Breaking your fast" is the term used when you consume any calories for the first time after a period of fasting, whether it's 12 hours or 24. However, there are many things you need to be careful of when it comes to breaking your fast. Making a mistake here could lead to severe stomach cramps, bloating, insulin overload, or constipation. You also need to be careful not to accidentally break your fast before it's time for it to be over.

That is, if you're doing a 16/8 style intermittent fast, consuming any calories 9 hours into the fasting period will immediately take you out of the fasting state, negating all your progress up to that point and sending you back to square one.

If you break your fast by immediately consuming a plate of pasta with a hearty dessert, your body is going to have some things to say about that. Going from no blood glucose to a full-blown insulin surge can fry your system for a while and make going into your fast again more challenging. You might also have to spend some time doubled over in pain, while your body processes the copious amount of inflammatory foods it just got loaded with. Certain high fiber foods are also not something to load up an empty stomach with since they'll be metabolized far faster than fibers should be.

It can be a good idea to break your fast with liquid so that you aren't overloading your empty stomach right off the bat. Bone broth, MCT or coconut oil, bulletproof coffee, or even a glass of non-dairy milk are ways that you can gently break your fast and stimulate your metabolic system just enough to be ready for some real food. Non-dairy mild is specified here because regular dairy has inflammatory properties, and even if that doesn't usually bother you, inflammation and an empty stomach do not mix. Keep in mind that if you have any of these drinks during your fast, even just a tiny bit, they will break your fast.

The reason that you're fasting or what changes you're hoping to see can help you determine what to break your fast with. Consuming certain foods first thing after a fasting period will help your body absorb more nutrients that are similar to your fast breaker.

If you're fasting for health-related reasons, bone broth is going to be the most ideal way to break your fast. It contains a generous amount of collagen, which helps strengthen your bones, cartilage, and is vital for stomach health. Anything you eat containing collagen after that point will be easily absorbed and fully utilized.

If you're looking for weight loss, MCT oil is an amazing way to break a fast, because the nutrients it contains pass directly into your stomach without hitting your liver first. This means that they will be utilized in your body very soon after consumption, and since it's fat with no carbs, you can break your fast without having any effect on your blood glucose. Consuming MCT oil to initially break your fast will also help your body properly utilize all the fats you put in during that eating period since you've just primed your stomach and metabolism with incredibly healthy fat.

After your stomach has something in it, you can break out the main courses. Whatever you would usually eat is fine at this point, in moderation. However, it is not a good idea to combine fats and carbohydrates while you are practicing an intermittent fast. That includes things like bread with butter, certain pastries, or pasta with butter or oil. The reason for this is that they have negative effects on your insulin and glucose levels when digested together, which is one of the major things you're trying to avoid while on this diet plan.

Carbohydrates trigger a significant rise in insulin and blood glucose, prompting your body to be much more absorbent of anything inside of it. Fats, by contrast, don't trigger any reaction from insulin if consumed without carbs.

But if they're combined and your cells are actively absorbing all the nutrients you're giving them, that is going to include the fats.

This translates to you adding more to your fat stores and basically resetting any process that may have been made during your last fasting period.

How Fasting Affects Your Body (You Aren't Dying)

TOP 10 INTERMITTENT FASTING MYTHS

- Unnatural and Unhealthy for the Body
- Slows Down Your Metabolism
- Causes Nutrient Deficiencies
- Causes Muscle Loss
- Leads to Eating Disorders
- Not Good For People with Diabetes
- Encourages Overeating
- You Shouldn't Exercise While Fasting
- You Will Feel Starved and Irritable
- It Will Cause Food Cravings

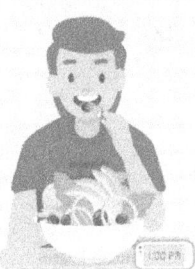

Let's really drive this home: the first three to five days of your fast are going to be the worst. You will feel hungry, tired, irritable, sluggish... but this is just your body trying to figure out what's going on. Once you have properly adjusted, these side effects will be significantly alleviated. You will still see some of the effects of consuming less calories, but once the positive benefits kick in, you'll feel a lot less like you're dying.

Feeling Unusually Cold

When you begin fasting, you'll notice that your fingers, hands, and maybe feet get a lot colder than usual, even if your fast is taking place in the summer. This will probably extend beyond the first few days, occurring regularly during all your fasting periods. Don't be worried, though; feeling cold while fasting is completely normal. In addition to your thyroid slowing down while you have low blood glucose, your body is also sending more blood flow to heat your core and fat stores, which pulls some blood flow from your extremities. And in general, having low blood sugar tend to make you more sensitive to the cold.

Countering this symptom is a lot easier than some of the others. Wearing more layers, sipping on hot tea or coffee, or hanging out outside on a summer day are some of the easiest ways. Exercises including yoga and light cardio can also be helpful. Whatever gets your blood flowing and your heart pounding will make you feel warm, at least until it's time to eat again.

This is something that you should monitor over time, however. If you feel cold even after exercise or eating a hearty meal, that could be a sign that there is damage to your thyroid or that it's working slower than it should be. In this case, there are tests that medical professionals can do to help you balance it back out.

Hunger

Unfortunately, there's almost no way around hunger at the beginning of your fast. It just takes some major willpower. The main reason that it's so hard to ebb your hunger at first is because your levels of ghrelin are still accustomed to your usual eating regimen, which is an average of three to six times a day. Every time you would usually have a meal, your ghrelin levels spike. This is out of memory, not necessity. Even though that doesn't make the gnawing hunger any easier to ignore, at least you know that you're on the right track to resetting your ghrelin. As long as you don't give in to hunger pangs, your ghrelin and related hormones will adapt to your new eating habits.

One way to help alleviate hunger is by drinking water almost excessively. Sparkling water, pH water, electrolyte water—so long as it doesn't have calories. This gives your stomach something to focus on while simultaneously giving your body something it needs. It may feel a little weird to have a stomach full of nothing but water, but at least it will quiet down for a while. Decaffeinated tea or coffee are also good for curbing the initial hunger pangs. Caffeinated is fine too, but it does boost your adrenal levels, which can speed up your metabolic processes, and that isn't too helpful in terms of tricking your hormones out of being hungry.

Another thing you'll notice in the face of this initial hunger is that your cravings for carbohydrates (sugary ones, like pastries) might go through the roof. This is your body looking for a quick blood glucose fix because they haven't started pulling from alternative sources yet. Once your cells start pulling their energy from sources like your fat cells, these excessive cravings should go back down to normal.

Headaches and Low Energy

These symptoms are common with general hunger and are to be expected when you start fasting. During the first few days, you may experience what most people describe as a dull, throbbing headache, and possibly muscle cramps as well. There are a few major causes of these, hunger being one, but also including dehydration, vitamin or electrolyte deficiency, and hormonal imbalances.

Stay hydrated. Reading that phrase will probably seem like listening to a broken record after a while, but it is one of the best things you can do for your body. Fasting or not, water and electrolytes are vital to your health and satiation. If you notice a headache setting in or your legs begin to ache, take that as your cue to have a glass of water, and maybe add some electrolytes or salt. These may not be all-encompassing cures to the initial discomfort of fasting, but they won't do anything but good for your body.

In terms of hormonal imbalances affecting your energy, that may be another thing that you have to ride out until your body adjusts. But as long as you adhere to a strict schedule during your intermittent fast, they should be able to balance out within the first few days.

Heartburn

This isn't as common as the other side effects, but it isn't unheard of. Your stomach produces acid to dige   st food, so when there is no food to digest, that could cause some discomfort. While not everyone experiences it, don't be alarmed if you experience heartburn during your fasting periods. It can certainly be painful and uncomfortable, but it is normal. Light doses of heartburn medication or sparkling water can help ease this symptom until you can eat again, at which point it should stop altogether.

If You'll Excuse Me...

Unfortunately, all those times that this book (and every medical professional) says to stay hydrated doesn't come without a price. And that price is how often you're going to need to use the bathroom.

With nothing in your stomach to absorb the liquid you put in, it's going to go straight through you. Adding electrolytes to your water might also help in this regard since it gives your body more to absorb, but it won't stop your bladder from doing its job, too. While using the restroom twice as much as usual might be unusual and inconvenient, just consider how uncomfortable you'd be otherwise. If you get dehydrated while you're fasting, it can lead to bloating, muscle cramps, and even constipation. It is much healthier to flush your body out a lot more than usual than it is to be unable to use the restroom at all.

Chapter 4:

Meal Planning & Menu Items

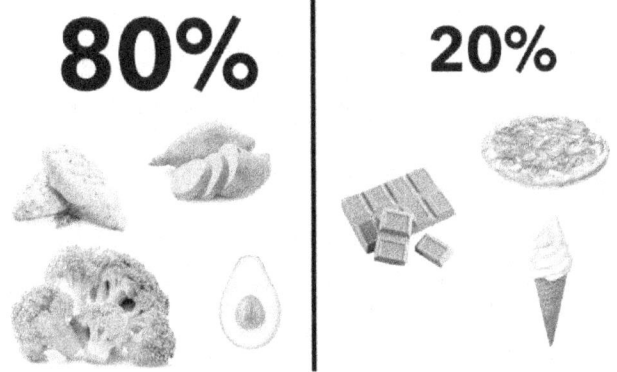

Unlike other weight loss plans, intermittent fasting is not highly restrictive about what you can, should, and can't eat. In the broadest sense, you can eat however much of whatever you like, so long as you only do so within the designated timeframes. With that in mind, this chapter isn't here to lay out any strict guidelines as other dietary books try to. Rather, it will explore how different diets interact with intermittent fasting, what foods you can eat (and how to prepare them) to optimize the benefits of the fast and explain what you might want to avoid eating in the case of certain health issues. Outside these recommendations, the only limitations you face with intermittent fasting are your own dietary needs and a tighter schedule.

In addition to being able to eat your favorite foods while fasting, it's significantly less expensive to do so. An intermittent fasting plan has the potential to help you save money. Although this component isn't as popular of a topic as the health benefits of intermittent fasting, it's still a notable perk. When you're budgeting in preparation for intermittent fasting, you can plan to buy the same foods that you usually would—but you'll only need about half the amount. And during the fasting window, the temptation to snag a treat from the gas station on your way home will, hopefully, be a lot less prominent. A lot of our snacking habits are centered around instant gratification, and if you know you have another 9 hours to go until you can eat again, that should negate some of the cravings for impulsively buying extra treats. Between that and not having an excuse to eat out as often, while you strive to lose weight during your fast, you might notice your wallet bulking up a bit.

Meal Planning

When it comes to planning your "meals," intermittent fasting makes things easier than almost any other diet. All you really need to plan is which routine you want to adhere to, choosing between 16/8, alternate day, or crescendo. From there, just eat like you normally would... but less often. If "breakfast time" occurs during your fasting period, then rejoice; you have the easiest, quickest breakfast options in the world. Grab a hot cup of coffee or tea and go about your day.

On an idealistic level, planning your meals for the day is the least stressful part of intermittent fasting. However, everyone's bodies and minds work differently and have different needs, so this might be easier said than done for some folks. Here are some quick pointers to keep in mind while trying to balance fasting, eating, and daily life.

Don't "Skip Meals"

Once the time rolls around for you to break your fast, it's a good idea to eat or drink something caloric as soon as possible. Your body will get used to eating once or twice a day, which is great—but that also means that if you're late to your first meal, the resulting hunger will be way more intense than you might be used to. While that's mostly your hormones talking, it's still uncomfortable and can have effects including nausea, irritability, or feeling intensely tired.

If you go into some days know that your busy schedule might hinder your ability to sit down for a meal on time, carrying light snacks or drinks—like juice or bone broth—is perfectly fine.

Don't be tempted have them before it's time to break your fast, though; just have them on hand in case breakfast isn't an option right away.

Balancing Social Situations

For a lot of people, going to a restaurant or bar with friends is the pinnacle of socializing. There's usually music, energizing atmosphere, and most importantly, great food and drinks. All of this is fun to experience with friends—unless you're actively fasting while everyone else has a plate of amazing food, in which case your glass of water or black coffee might seem a little bleak.

If you and your friends, family, or partner go out on a regular basis, it's a good idea (for you, at least), only to go out during your eating period. That way you can enjoy the environment and commodities just as much as everybody else. If you're in a fasted state and your social circle wants to hang out, suggest something less food-oriented, like seeing a movie or bowling. While there might not be any rules about not being near food while in a fasted state, it can definitely challenge your willpower in an uncomfortable way to be literally surrounded by food and people eating.

Worry about Nutrition—Not Calories

While on an intermittent fast, it's especially important to pack more nutrients onto your plate than usual, because you have less time —and therefore, less opportunity—each day to get all your vital nutrients.

As you read before, when planning what you're going to eat for the day, foods with fats, vitamins, and proteins should be on your mind before carbs and sugar.

Eating a healthy far during each meal will be great for your body and metabolic functions, and it will also keep cravings at bay. If you get enough fats and vitamins in during your eating window, you'll feel satiated for much longer into your fasted state.

The last thing you need to do on an intermittent fast is count calories. As Dr. Jason Fung said, calories have next to no bearing on our weight and metabolic processes. What does matter is what you are eating. 500 "calories" worth of salad and vegetables is going to be much better for you in every way that the equivalent amount of pastries or candy bars. Foods that are packed with nutrition and don't send your blood glucose sky-high are not only better for you, but they won't leave your feeling dissatisfied and hungry in an hour. Healthy foods stick with you for much longer than sugary, empty calories.

Ketogenic Intermittent Fasting

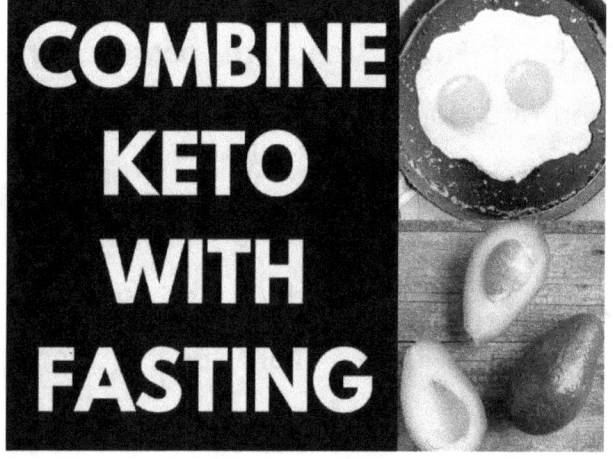

Ketogenic diet restrictions and intermittent fasting are one of the most popular power couples in the world of dieting. They compliment each other extremely well; fasting increases ketosis, and ketosis can amplify the effects of the rest of your fast. Combining an intermittent fast with a ketogenic diet is more challenging and restrictive, but certainly not without strong benefits.

A pinnacle guideline in the Keto diet is to drastically reduce your carb intake, nearly to the point of elimination. As a result, your general insulin levels are also decreased. And in an intermittent fast, you are eating much less frequently, which also leads to reduced insulin levels. With both keto and fasting having amazing insulin-reducing effects, the combination of the two can alleviate issues such as insulin resistance, inflammation, and lethargy.

Basic Keto Guidelines

The keto diet works by, in a way, flipping around the food pyramid that we're used to seeing in classrooms and doctor's offices. While our standard food pyramid has grains as one of the most consumed items and oils and fats at the very tip, the ketogenic diet almost entirely eradicated grains and carbohydrates, while natural fats make up a large portion of the diet's base.

In the ideal percentage breakdown for the keto diet, 75% of your energy should be coming from natural fats, 15–25% should be coming from protein, and <5% should be coming from carbohydrates. 0% should come from sugar. The lesser carbohydrates, the better. For a lot of people, this can be rough at first. After all, glucose and carbs have become our most defaulted to sources of energy. It takes out bodies time to make the switch to relying on ketones instead. But as it is with intermittent fasting, the longer you go without sugar and carbs, the less your body will actively crave them.

Keto practitioners usually see a very basic assortment of foods in their diet.

These include natural fats and oils (butter, dairy, coconut oil, etc.), eggs, meat, fish, vegetables that grow above ground (root vegetables are higher in carbohydrates), and some fruit.

Foods to generally be avoided during keto are most fruits (since their sugar content is high), candy of any kind, beer, juice, and soda, refined carbohydrates (bread, pastries, pasta), root vegetables, and rice.

Keto is so different from how most of us are used to eating because the starchy foods that have become our default dietary staples of the years are not allowed. This is similar to the Paleo diet, with the main differences being the energy percentage breakdown, and that many processed foods are keto-friendly. But otherwise, the two diets are very much alike.

Disclaimer for Keto + Fasting

If you are not currently on a ketogenic diet, trying to go full keto at the same time as starting an intermittent fast could have some severe effects on your wellbeing. At the start of both keto and fasting, you may experience flu-like symptoms like shakes, coldness, nausea, and consistently not having energy. Beginning both of these plans at the same time could send your body into a full sickness, rather than just showing the symptoms of one. However, if you are definitely interested in trying keto and seeing if it works for you, there are some things you can try.

If the ketogenic diet seems like a better choice for your dietary needs and weight loss goals but you still want to try intermittent fasting, then the crescendo fast might be the best option for you. This way, you can fully commit to a ketogenic diet, and try fasting a few days out of the week to see how it affects you. On a keto diet, even with only a few days of intermittent fasting, you'll see some amazing benefits in terms of weight loss, muscle gain, and mental clarity. The sugar and carb craving will be gnarly, but at least not as bad as they would be if you tried both diet plans at once.

Another option would be to go the other way around: fully implement your intermittent fast and try eating exclusively keto foods a few days a week. You could also try one or two ketogenic meals a day in combination with your regular food, but you would have to be very careful with this approach. Eating carbs and a keto meal on the same day not only negate most of the keto's effects but it can also have negative effects, as you would be consuming both fats and carbohydrates. To that end, it may just be easier to set aside one or two days a week to be your "keto" days.

In that approach, you would be able to see very, very accurately what the differences between your current diet and a ketogenic one would be. During your fasting periods, your body has time to metabolize all the food you ate in your last eating window. If you ate a strictly ketogenic meal after 16 hours of fasting, you would most likely notice the differences immediately and more accurately than you would by just trying out keto during a regular eating schedule. This can be a great method to see if keto is truly a diet you want to pursue, or if you'll be content just sticking with intermittent fasting.

Powerful Anti-inflammatory & Antioxidant Meal Plans

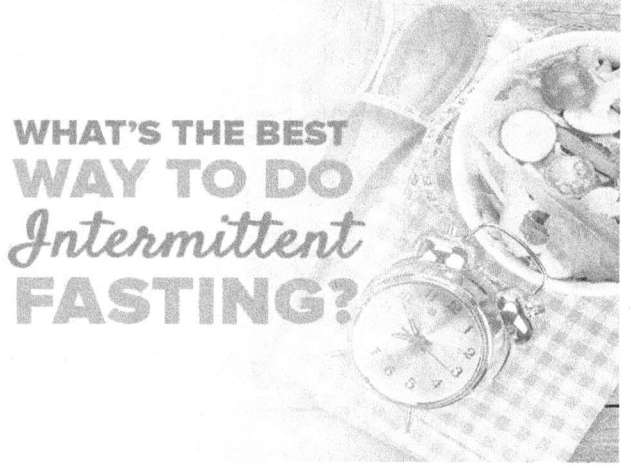

While intermittent fasting in a powerful weapon against chronic inflammation in and of itself, adding anti-inflammatory foods into your daily routine can amplify these benefits. The same goes for foods high in antioxidants. By including foods that pack a nutritional punch against potential issues to your diet, you will see some of the intermittent fasting's perks optimized.

Foods That Cause Inflammation

Unfortunately, many foods that we regularly consume day-to-day have severe effects on inflammation and pain in our bodies. Evolutionarily speaking, we aren't accustomed to consuming highly processed foods and copious amounts of sugar. Since you'll be eating less in general during your intermittent fast and more time to plan your meals, it introduces a good opportunity to practice cutting out some of the worst offenders to inflammation.

Refined grains and sugars, or food with a high-glycemic index, are some of the most inflammation inducing things you can consume. Many, many kinds of processed foods fit into this category. As you read in Chapter 2, a diet high in these types of food can lead to increased blood glucose, insulin resistance, and even prediabetes. During the eating periods of an intermittent fast, you might consider abstaining from refined grains like pasta, pastries, and white bread, and foods that are high in sugar. This will not only decrease your overall inflammations but will also allow autophagy and insulin sensitivity to see an increase.

Foods that are high in omega-6 fatty acids can also contribute to your body's overall inflammation. These include dairy products, red meat, and vegetable oils. Omega-6 is important to your overall health, so you shouldn't cut it out altogether—but in excess, it can be harmful. In an anti-inflammatory diet, you can still eat dairy products and meat if you choose, just in careful moderation. During an intermittent fast these should pose significantly less of a problem, due to your overall decrease in all foods.

Anti-inflammatory Foods

Studies have shown that antioxidizing foods and those that are high in omega-3 fatty acids (fish) have incredible anti-inflammatory properties. Since inflammation can be caused by oxidative stress or high levels of insulin, eating foods that combat these issues can help with inflammation by proxy. These are foods that are not only powerful accomplices to the intermittent fasting plan but are also delicious, accessible and easy to include in your daily life.

Berries of all sorts—blueberries, blackberries, strawberries—are all amazing sources of antioxidants. Nuts, dark leafy greens, and beans also fit this profile. There's also broccoli, apples, avocados... anything high in healthy fiber, fats, and vitamins can usually claim some antioxidizing or anti-inflammatory benefits as well. The list of anti-inflammatory foods is surprisingly long and full of variety.

If you're worried about keeping inflammation in check after your intermittent fast has run its course, it is not unreasonable to look into maintaining an exclusively anti-inflammatory diet. There are many guides and books available on this idea since inflammation is such a strong cause of distress in our modern lives. Some diets are even anti-inflammatory by default, including paleo and keto. Just keep in mind: the worst offenders for inflammation are sugars and refined grains, while nutrient-rich and antioxidizing foods are powerful tools to fight against it.

Vegan Intermittent Fasting

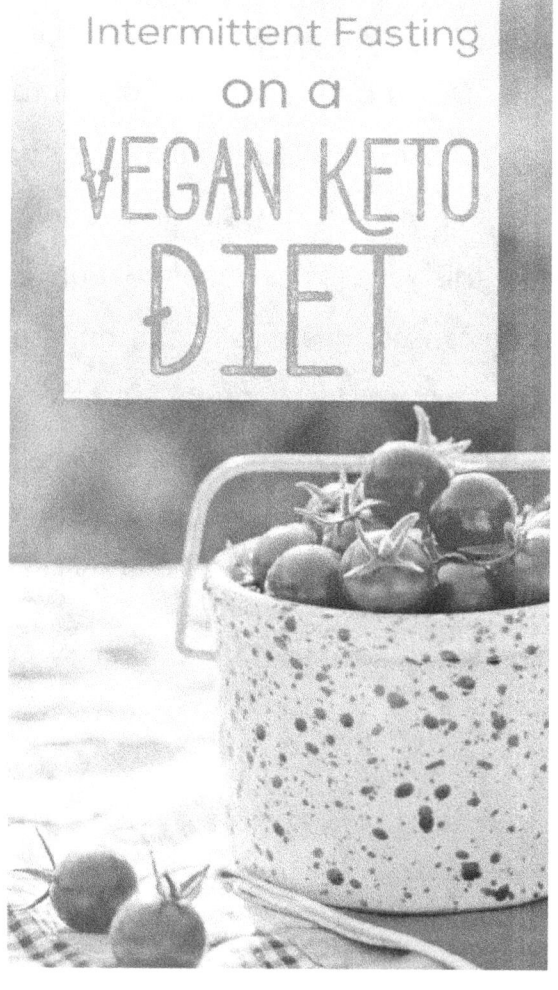

Engaging in an intermittent fasting lifestyle as a vegan is arguably easier to accomplish than being vegan on a normal eating schedule. This ties into the fact that intermittent fasting can be a catalyst saving money. Many (healthy) vegan foods and resources are not cheap, and there is also a significant amount of food marketed towards vegans that are full of empty calories, unhealthy levels of soy, or so processed that they are nearly void of nutrients.

As a vegan on an intermittent fasting regimen, it can be easier to save money not only because you need to eat less often, but because it can be easier to eat raw or fresh foods more frequently. Stockpiling fresh fruits and vegetables can easily become the equivalent of throwing away money if you don't eat them fast enough because they go bad much more quickly than processed foods.

This becomes a nasty pitfall for a lot of vegans, as they turn to processed meals and less nutritious options that have a longer shelf life. But if you only need to worry about one or two meals a day, it can be a lot cheaper to just buy produce as you need it (if you live within a close distance of a grocery store.)

While the foods in this section are vegan (contain no animal products or byproducts), that does not take away from the advantage of adding some of them to your daily routine. Getting fruits, vegetables, and greens on your plate while fasting is one of the most important and performance-enhancing things you can do. Even if you are a devout meat eater who might take a small salad with your steak every once and a while, these foods are worth considering based on their powerful antioxidizing, anti-inflammatory, and fat burning capabilities.

Salads

If you're not used to eating salads, an intermittent fasting lifestyle might be a great excuse for you to try incorporating them daily, at least as a snack. Salads can be a blast to make and experiment with, especially if you know what health benefits you're trying to gain from eating them. As a bonus, most ingredients that you would usually have on a salad can be bought in bulk, like nuts and dried fruit. Have fun with combining flavors and toppings and enjoy the added benefits that they add to your health and your fast.

For any salad base, you should focus on dark leafy greens. Most spring mixes have a great variety. Arugula, spinach, and kale are also nutrient power-houses that can be added to any salad (or meal in general) to add an extra punch of vitamins.

Anti-inflammatory Salad Toppings

If your objective is to fight inflammation as you continue fasting, some of these salad toppings would be wonderful to try. Some of the best contenders include beets, fresh berries, nuts (almonds, walnuts, pecans, hazelnuts), avocado, broccoli, apples, cherries, beans (red, pinto, or black), artichoke hearts, olives, shredded coconut, and cauliflower.

High Protein Salad Toppings

Every vegan has probably heard "But how do you get your protein?" at some point during their diet. Here are some easy answers to that question that also happens to taste great with salad: tofu and edamame (soy protein), nutritional yeast, almost all beans, green peas, quinoa, spinach, artichokes, all nuts, and chia seeds.

Antioxidizing Salad Toppings

There's a lot of overlap with other benefits here, so many of these will look familiar. Some of the best are goji berries, blueberries, walnuts, pecans, grapes, and turmeric. These are also helpful for improving autophagy.

Combinations to Try

For protein power:

- Spinach, artichokes, shredded almonds, walnuts, quinoa or chia seeds (or both, but the texture might be extra gritty), black beans, tofu (or hardboiled eggs for nonvegans)

For fruit lovers:

- Spring mix, blueberries, sliced strawberries, shredded almonds, goji berries, apple chunks, orange slices, cherries, and poppy seed dressing

For fighting inflammation:

- Spinach, kale, parsley, pickled beets, kidney beans, broccoli, nutritional yeast, artichoke hearts, and a creamy avocado dressing

Southwest style spice:

- Spring mix, arugula, cilantro, bell pepper, black and red beans, turmeric, smoked corn, onion and tomato

Healthy Snacks to Keep You Going

Don't confuse this section with how you may think of snacking now. "Snacks" can still only be had during your eating window, so that doesn't leave a lot of time for grazing. However, there are some very delicious smaller fare foods that can help keep you satiated and your blood sugar level for longer into the fasting window. Since easy snacks to make yourself usually consist of only a few ingredients, there is plenty to go around for every diet and meal plan.

While you're on an intermittent fasting plan, experimenting with food (even just lighter fare snacks) during your eating window can be a nice way to give yourself a change of pace from your usual eating habits. Try out some of these snacks, either to take to work, share with guests, or just play around in the kitchen for a bit. There are a plethora of fun and easy combinations and recipes you can try. And variety is something that's always nice to have, especially if you're new to a restrictive diet like keto and worried about missing out on foods.

The important things to remember if you do experiment with meal or snack recipes is not to combine fats and carbs. Eating that combination specifically within the same eating window can be detrimental to your blood glucose, as well as how much fat you might absorb. For increased natural ketosis, you should go with fats; for an extra boost for your blood glucose, carbs are the way to go.

You might also avoid adding sugar to things in general. Plenty of treats contain fruits and other ingredients that contain natural sugars, so you should lean on these to replace refined, added sugar. If a recipe calls for sugar, then add it—just not an excessive amount. It's important to work with your body while you're fasting. If you consume sugar during every eating window, you won't be doing yourself any favors in terms of curbing carb cravings in the long run.

Here are some examples of appetizers, snacks, and light-fare courses that you can try during your eating window. The ingredients here are just suggestions; if you're following specific dietary restrictions, most of these are flexible and can be modified accordingly. Feel free to make your own combinations, too. You might find something healthy and delicious that you want to keep in your diet even after your fast.

Fried Rice

This is one of the more malleable options, working great as either a snack or the base of a meal. Usually, fried rice consists of white or brown rice, peas, carrots, green onions, and egg. Since rice is a hefty carbohydrate, you should make sure not to make/buy fried rice with butter or excessive oil. Instead, use soy sauce or the seasoning of your choice to help with the dry texture. To make an anti-inflammatory meal centered around fried rice, add a fillet of salmon and a side of steamed vegetables.

Steamed Broccoli

Broccoli in any form is healthy, as long as you don't have too much. It's especially great to have while on an intermittent fast since it's so dense with nutrients. Steaming it gives it a softer texture, without losing too many nutrients to water like boiling it would.

For an added boost, you can add salt and a bit of coconut oil or cheese (dairy or soy) once it's steamed. The salt will keep your sodium electrolytes balanced, and the healthy fats from the coconut oil or cheese will keep you satiated for longer without increasing your blood glucose.

Miso Soup

A popular appetizer in Asian style restaurants, miso soup has a surprising amount of health benefits and not a lot of calories. It's a pescatarian (sometimes vegetarian) option, usually made with fish broth, seaweed, bits of tofu, green onion, and soy sauce. With the broth and small amount of protein from tofu, miso soup can be a great way to break your fast if you're looking for something new.

Hardboiled Eggs

A classic, easy snack if you're on the go or just short on time. Boil a dozen at the beginning of your week and you'll have something quick to grab if you're running out the door. Again, add salt to get your electrolytes up. One hardboiled egg has about 70 calories and a generous amount of protein. If you're on a ketogenic diet, this is a great snack to have on hand during your eating window.

Baked Apples with Cinnamon

This one is almost too easy... and so good. Core an apple, cut it into wedges, glaze them with cinnamon, clove, cardamom, or whatever other spice you've got a hankering for (not sugar) and put it in the oven for 5-10 minutes.

While apples are packed with vitamins and fiber, spices like cinnamon can help stabilize blood sugar levels and curb sugar cravings. Plus, it's delicious.

Air Pop Popcorn

Air popped popcorn has limitless possibilities. On a ketogenic diet? Add a hearty splash of melted butter, or coconut oil if you can't have dairy. Looking for some spice? Mix in some cayenne, black peppercorn, and salt. Want a snack on the sweeter side? Combine melted butter, dark chocolate chips and/or cinnamon, and a dash of salt. With the right combination of spices, you can have a snack similar to those which you might find at a gas station... but significantly healthier.

Frozen Blueberries

It doesn't get easier than this. Blueberries are a good source of antioxidants as well as satisfyingly, naturally sweet. Have a small bowl on hand to snack on as a replace for candy or chips, or just to add a little extra variety to your snacking experience. Add them to oatmeal or whole grain cereals to add extra flavor and nutrients. They're great to add to meals, or just to graze on. Fresh blueberries are equally delicious—they just tend to have a much shorter shelf life.

Dark Chocolate

As long as it's at least 70% dark chocolate, then this popular dessert actually has some great health benefits. Dark chocolate has impressive antioxidant and anti-inflammatory properties.

Be careful of which kind you buy, as many dark chocolates have a lot of added sugar— but as long as there isn't an excessive amount, feel free to welcome this treat into your diet. Melt it fondue-style and dip berries and fruit slices in or put a chunk or two in hot water or milk and stir for improvised hot chocolate. Dark chocolate, high sugar or not, might improve mood and stabilize blood glucose, so if you need a pick me up a snack after a long day, dark chocolate is there for you.

Chapter 5:

Self Care Tips—Staying Healthy & Active While Fasting

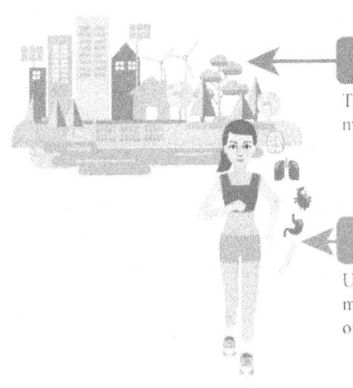

Metabolic Flexibility

The ability to change our metabolism to meet the demands of our environment.

Energy Efficiency

Using our energy in the most efficient matter possible to regulate all the needs of the body.

Aside from being a new way of eating, intermittent fasting involves making some major changes to your general lifestyle. In addition to being faced with hunger, sugar cravings, and hormonal changes at the start of your fast, you'll also hit some hurdles when it comes to your subconscious habits and activities. For example, eating out of boredom or stress is something that not a lot of thought goes in to beforehand—and could ruin the effects of your fast in an instant. Social interactions have subliminal effects on our eating habits as well. Even just running to the store for paper towels can influence your thoughts and actions in terms of food.

The aim of this chapter will be to help you break old habits and create new ones. While life-long mannerisms may be comfortable to slip in to at first, you will notice a significant difference in your energy, mood, and mobility by breaking unhealthy habits in favor of ones that center around your health while fasting. We will explore how marketing and advertisements can be a conduit for overeating and health issues, and how to rewire your brain to ignore them. The tips and tricks in this chapter are centered around the intermittent fasting lifestyle, but even outside of the fasting plan, they can be powerful ways to enhance your quality of life.

Jingles, Sugar, & Other Reasons You Can't Stop Eating

It can be extremely difficult to just "eat less," or even less often, in our modern society. Most of us can walk a few blocks to the nearest gas station for a pick-me-up snack or pay someone else to drive food to our own house. In urban America, food is arguably one of the most accessible resources available to us.

Food and food services make up one of the most advertised, capitalized industries... and one of the most addictive ones.

Companies whose profit comes from mainly foods are completely aware of how effective their advertising is. Kids' food is packaged in bright, cartoony, fun containers to draw attention, and for more grown-up appeal, things like "low carbs!" or "certified gluten-free!" are printed broadly on way more foods than necessary. If the packaging is eye-catching, more consumers are likely to hurriedly toss it in their carts. Bright packaging that advertises exactly what dietary restrictions we might need mitigates the stress of searching the other choices and gets us out of the store more quickly... but not without spending more money than we might have.

With shopping aside, how many times have you (or your children, roommates, or friends) heard the jingle of a popular fast food chain and immediately gotten a hankering for a burger and fries? Again—companies know exactly how effective they can trigger our innate food cravings with their advertisements. Our associating with food is very strong since it's such a vital part of our everyday lives. We see food industries all over the place, too, from televised commercials to driving past blocks of back-to-back fast food joints on the way to work. It's everywhere.

The general accessibility we have to food is a great testament to how far we've come as a first world country—and how effectively companies can get public masses addicted to their products.

A dirty little secret that almost all food manufacturers utilize is that they add sugar to nearly all their products, sweet or not. Why? Sugar keeps you coming back.

If you check the ingredients, even foods like pasta, savory sauces, and hamburger buns have some amount of added sugar. There is a marketing term know as the "bliss point," which denotes the method of adding sugar to bland, spicy, or otherwise savory foods until just barely below the point where it would be considered "sweet." When we eat foods that are at or just below the "bliss point," especially if they are heavy in carbohydrates, it tricks our pancreas into way overshooting the amount of insulin it needs to produce. By the time our cells have absorbed the blood glucose that we just consumed, there is still an excessive amount of insulin left in our bloodstream. With nothing to do and nowhere to go, it starts calling for another job to do.

Having excess insulin makes us feel hungry much, much faster than we would be otherwise. Consequentially, we tend to consume a lot more foods with added sugars than we reasonably need to. This can lead to insulin resistance, detrimental sugar cravings, and weight gain—but also leads us to buy more of the product we're craving. And companies have figured this out, so why not add sugar to inconspicuous products to keep us hungry for more?

How & Why to Cut Refined Sugar Consumption

One of the primary reasons we crave sugar so fervently is because it activates the part of our brain that induces pleasure and happiness.

So even if we understand the negative effects of sugar on our overall health, it may be hard to get out of the mindset of "it makes me feel good, so why should I stop?" Your brain, as we've explored, is as closely tied to your cravings and hunger as the rest of your hunger hormones, so this is a pretty compelling internal argument.

During an intermittent fast, try cutting your refined sugar consumption down as much as possible during your eating window. Sugar alternatives in moderation can be a great way to help you cut your cravings. Stevia is an especially good one to combine with an intermittent fast because it doesn't spike your blood glucose or trigger insulin release like other sugar alternatives—and it isn't artificial. Cinnamon is also a wonderful spice to add to coffee, teas, and meals to curb sugar cravings, along with multiple other health benefits. And if you absolutely need to, add a light amount of honey to things for extra sweetness. While honey is heavy in sugar, it also has actual health benefits that pure refined sugar does not.

When you intentionally cut down on your sugar intake, even without fasting, you'll notice a general decrease in energy dips and mood swings between meals/snacks. Cutting sugar makes your blood glucose spikes less extreme and can also improve your sensitivity to insulin. Try not to listen to your brain for the first few days when it's crying for sugar; after your body recognizes how good you feel with less sugar in your system, sugar cravings should naturally subside, making the whole process of cutting sugar easier from there.

Cutting sugar, and reducing sugar cravings by proxy, can also help you become more aware of what your body is actually craving. Sweets and carbs won't be your default craving once your stomach starts growling, so you'll have a more acute sense of what nutrients your body is needing at the moment. Protein, potassium, water, and salts are all things that your body might be craving, but that your brain usually overrides with "More sugar, please."

Sugar Alternatives & Their Benefits

This isn't to say that your diet should be void of anything sweet. Refined sugar may be full of empty calories, but there are a surprising among of delicious, sweet alternatives to sugar that can actually be beneficial to your health. Some of them are even sweeter than sugar and don't raise your blood glucose nearly as much.

Raw honey is by far one of the most popular sugar alternatives. It's doesn't spike blood glucose nearly as much as sugar, has antioxidizing properties, and even contains some electrolytes. It's also considered a whole food, and raw honey is never artificial. Honey also has one incredibly unique element: if you're consuming honey from anywhere near your local area, the pollen it contains can help build immunity to certain allergens that are common around you.

Another whole food sugar alternative is dates. These are high in fiber and potassium, which is definitely something that refined sugar cannot claim. Rather than making you feel bloated and even constipated, the nutrients in dates can help to... keep things moving. Dates are even more malleable than honey; many paleo or gluten-free power bars use dates as their base, since their consistency is thick and hold together so well. Their use in snack foods like power bars and candies is a testament to how well dates' flavor melds with other foods, especially sweet ones.

Date syrup also exists and can be used in place of refined sugar in some recipes and is a delicious additive to black coffee. It can also be used as a cheaper alternative than pure maple syrup on breakfast foods—but an exponentially healthier choice than completely artificial "maple syrup."

Like dates, coconut sugar also contains potassium—and magnesium and prebiotic fibers. Coconut sugar is an awesome source for electrolytes, so if you're worried about getting enough in your diet and also looking for ways to control your blood glucose, throw away your refined sugar and bring in some coconut sugars. On its own or in coffee, you might notice a taste difference—but in more complex recipes, like pastries or smoothies, all you'll be able to notice is the added sweetness.

The last major sugar alternative is agave nectar, and it also happens to be an extremely popular one (although most people know it for tequila and not as a sweetener). Agave has interesting health benefits as well, including anti-inflammation and regulating digestion. It's very easy for your body to break down, and it's sweet in all the right ways; it doesn't send your blood glucose through the roof, but it contains enough natural sugar to give you a steady boost in energy and metabolic functions.

Supplements to Give You an Edge

As long as they don't contain calories or carbs, herbal and mineral supplements can be great resources to draw out more benefits from your fast, as well as make the process easier for your body.

Supplements that improve mood, curb sugar craving, increase energy and metabolic functions, or increase mineral absorption are all great ones to explore, both while fasting and while eating regularly. Aside from drawing out the benefits of your diet or fast, these supplements can greatly improve your quality of life.

An important note is that you should only take supplements with water during your fast, in order to improve how much your body absorbs. It's also fine to take them with food during your eating period. But taking supplements in combination with caffeinated teas or coffees nullifies a significant amount of the potential absorption, because thanks to the caffeine, you'll end up losing a lot of it to frequent urination.

Sodium, Magnesium, & Potassium

These are the most vital electrolytes that your body needs to function. Potassium is important for blood flow and heart functions, and sodium can prevent cramps and achiness. Magnesium has also been shown to help with the absorption of other minerals—so it might help to take a magnesium supplement during your first meal of the day.

Common complains during the start of a fast are headaches, body aches and muscle cramps, nausea, and heart palpitations. And usually, when you begin fasting, your body sees a general decline in vital electrolytes, because you're consuming less foods that contain them.

Adding any combination of these (or a comprehensive electrolyte supplement) can greatly ease these symptoms and improve the overall quality of your fast.

It is also recommended to increase your sodium intake while fasting to 15–18 g. (or 3 tsp.) a day.

Zinc

Zinc is an amino acid that helps insulin and glucose function at maximum capacity. By default, it also helps improve insulin sensitivity and balance blood sugar. Take a small dose of zinc every other day while fasting can help improve your insulin levels and assist in cutting cravings for carbs and sugar.

Vitamin B

A powerful source of vitamin B is nutritional yeast, which can be taken as a supplement or added to foods. Vitamin B can help reduce fatigue, as well as the flu-like symptoms and physical "heaviness" that often accompany switching to keto or intermittent fasting.

Turmeric & Curcumin

Turmeric and curcumin (a powerful extract derived from the turmeric plant) are incredible anti-inflammatory supplements. They have also been shown to help boost the effects of autophagy. By taking either of these as a supplement while fasting, you could radically increase intermittent fasting's anti-inflammatory benefits as well as giving autophagy a boost. These are also good supplements to take outside of fasting, as they can help promote energy and reduce inflammation and pain caused by the things we might not think about, like foods or working out incorrectly.

Exercising While You Fast

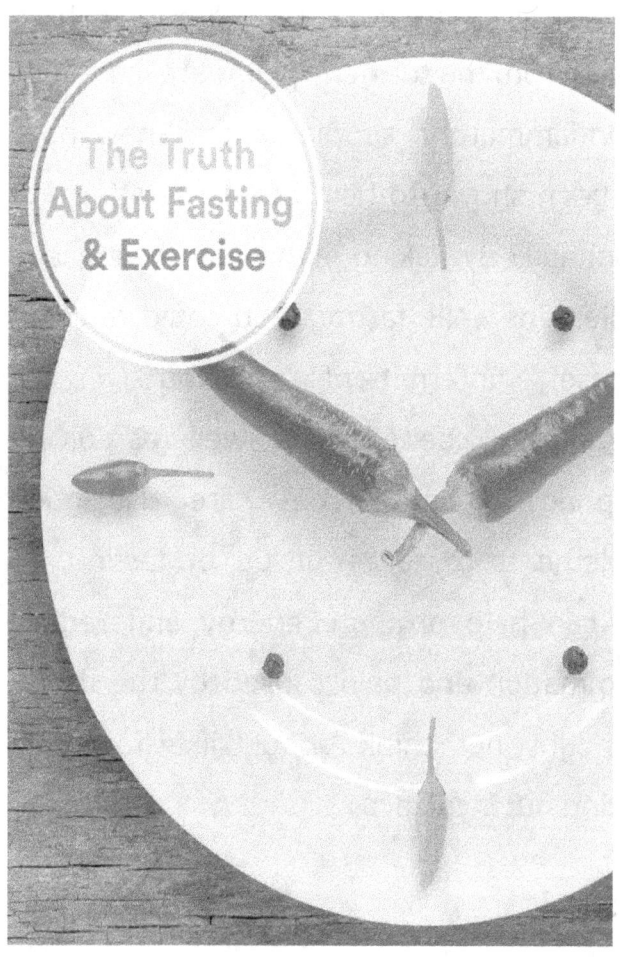

Just like there are multiple methods to engage in fasting, there isn't one set in stone recommendation for an exercise routine. How and when you exercise during a fast is entirely up to you, your body, and your comfort. If you're just in it for the autophagy and insulin sensitivity, you probably won't need to worry much about a rigorous workout schedule. If you're in it for the weight loss and muscle gain, this is probably the section you've been waiting for.

If regular workouts aren't already a part of your daily routine, then hitting the gym immediately after you begin your fast probably isn't the best idea. Your body is already going to be reeling from your sudden change in eating patterns; it's best not to add a new exercise routine into the mix right away. Just continue with your life as you usually would for the first few days and see how your mind and body are feeling.

Once you can feel that your body is adjusting to the fast, such as feeling hungry only during your new eating period and regaining your energy, then it's safer to implement new routines. Starting slow, of course, is ideal. If the adjustment period is taking you a bit longer, you can still exercise—but start with ease, mobility-oriented yoga or light cardio. These will get you moving and your blood flowing, and from there you can work up to more intense regimens.

When to Workout & Why

Like many other components in intermittent fasting, this doesn't have a universal answer.

It depends on your comfort and physical abilities, and you also have to take into consideration that working out at different points during your fast will yield different results.

If you stick with cardio as your main form of exercise, working out while you are in a fasted state can greatly improve the visible results. Like you read earlier, when you are in a fasted state, your blood flow is pulled away from your extremities and focuses more on your core and your fat stores. A major fat store that most people have is in their stomach. When you are fasting, the blood flow to your belly fat is significantly increased—which can exponentially increase the fat-burning impacts of fasted cardio exercises.

With that being said, exercising in a fasted state without previous experience doing so can be tricky, and timing it correctly makes a big difference on how you'll feel afterwards. There are multiple ways to do this: before you eat, right after you have your last meal, or in the middle of your fasting window. Exercising at the tail end of your fast (right before your first meal) may yield the best results for fat loss via cardio, because that is when the blood flow to your midsection will be going strong, and you'll have the added benefits of significantly increased human growth hormone and sympathetic nervous system engagement.

Those two factors—human growth hormones and sympathetic nervous system—are a major part of why some bodybuilders swear by the combination of exercise and fasting to improve the results of both. Fasting, as you read in chapter 1, is a strong enough stressor that doing it for extended periods of time triggers the stimulation of these and our norepinephrine.

These are all main components in our fight or flight response and fasting induces them because our body is trying to prepare us for danger and help us "find food."

So, what makes exercise and fasting such a powerful combination? Among other things: intensive exercise also stimulates human growth hormones and the sympathetic nervous system. Combining these leads to double the stimulation, a continuous rush of survival-driven energy, a powerful boost to adrenaline, and because of all this, increased fat loss and muscle gain. Part of the increase in fat loss is because with all these factors together, any lipids that have been stored in your muscles are getting rapidly flushed out in a way that regular exercise wouldn't do. Another factor is just how much raw energy you have during a fasted workout state. In addition to mental acuity, you might also feel ready to run a marathon—for a few minutes.

Timing your workout can be tricky. For people on a 16/8 plan or a variation thereof, there are two main times when they might workout: right before eating for the first time, or right after their last meal of the day. If the meal you're skipping is breakfast, you could work in an exercise routine first thing when you wake up, and then have your first meal a few hours after winding down. If your eating window is earlier in the day you could try a workout regimen right before hitting the hay. Working out prior to eating optimizes fat burning; working out after can increase energy and muscle gain. Either way, the unique benefits of fasting and exercise on your body and energy will be noticeable.

Folks trying out alternate day fasting may need to be a bit more careful when it comes to energy expenditure while fasting.

Since this plan involves 24 hours of fasting with no more than 500 calories, you'll be stretching the time you go without food by quite a few more hours. If you do a hardy workout first thing on your fasting day, you risk burning yourself out for the rest of the day. Ideal methods for exercising on this plan are either working out intensively right before going to bed on your fasting day or saving intensive exercise for your eating day and sticking to light cardio while you fast.

A crescendo fast is possibly the easiest method to go for if you're new to both workouts and fasting. On fasting day, it's best to stick to light cardio and yoga rather than intensive exercise. This will keep you moving, improving fat burning and autophagy, but it won't be nearly as taxing. On the days in this diet where you're eating regularly, starting a flexible workout regimen can be beneficial.

Implementing New Daily Rituals

Beginning an intermittent fast can be a major lifestyle change. If you aren't used to following a strict eating schedule, this might make the transition more difficult. Before you fast, and during the start of your new diet plan, it can be helpful to add new rituals and routines to your daily life. If you have a personal schedule to work your fasting routine around, you'll have less risk of forgetting when to beginning fasting or breaking your fast too early.

Morning Routine

We all have a set of rituals that we go through every morning, no matter how trivial the tasks may seem. These might include brushing our teeth, having breakfast, checking out social media... whatever you do on a daily basis when you get out of bed is a daily ritual. Be careful once you start fasting—if breakfast is no longer within your eating window (i.e. if you can't start eating until 2PM), you might be exceptionally hungry for the first few mornings. Skipping a daily ritual will really confuse your body for a few days. This can make it difficult to find energy, cause irritability, or make it feel like your day is dragging by.

Waking up at the same time each day can be immensely beneficial, whether you are fasting or not. If you tend to oversleep or don't get enough sleep regularly, this can affect many aspects of your fast. A lack of sleep is a stressor on your body, which is why folks with insomnia may want to be wary of intermittent fasting. Additionally, studies have shown that a sporadic sleep schedule can have the same effects on your body and mind as jet lag, making you feel more tired and sluggish than you would be otherwise.

When you start your intermittent fast, it would be worth your while to try going to sleep and waking up at around the same times each day. Not only will this help optimize the benefits of your sleep, but it will also help your body learn the new eating routine. Your internal clock isn't set on a 24 regimen like the ones we're used to seeing. If you usually eat 2 hours after you wake up, then your ghrelin levels will kick in, surprise, 2 hours after you wake up— regardless of whether you woke up at 7AM or noon. The situation will be the same once your body has adjusted to intermittent fasting. If you wake up at wildly different times each morning, you may feel excruciatingly hungry well before it's time to eat, or not hungry at all when the time comes, missing out on a portion of your eating window. Neither of these situations is ideal for your body or mind.

Every morning when you wake up, put the kettle on for tea. This one can be a lot easier than adjusting your sleep patterns. Once you wake up, check your phone, turn on the kettle, use the restroom. It's a minor addition to what you're probably used to already. Even if you're a devout coffee connoisseur, a cup of tea each morning can be extremely beneficial to your fast. As we've explored, green teas will assist in the autophagy and antioxidant processes of your body, while black teas will give you a smooth rush of energy from their caffeine content.

Herbal teas will help keep you satiated, and also have the potential to improve mood and aid in relaxation, as is the case with lavender or chamomile. A cup of hot tea every morning can be a nice replacement to breakfast, give you something to wash back medication with, and give your stomach something to work with that doesn't break your fast.

You can also try practicing some light cardio or yoga each morning. This gets your blood flowing, which can increase energy, help you shake off the fogginess of sleep, and can help with the coldness that accompanies the fasting period. Gently stimulating your muscles and joints in the morning can help you throughout the day as well, making you feel lighter, reducing muscle aches in the case of unexpected exercise (like if you have to run to catch the bus), and improving the fat burning effects of the fast. For people who want to see a decent amount of fat-burning effects from their fast but don't have time to hit the gym each day, cardio and yoga are a great, quick way to stimulate and improve the process. These exercises also have life-long benefits, such as prevention from mobility hindering issues like arthritis, and improved insulin sensitivity.

During the Day

Life is busy. Public transit, traffic jams, trouble at work, and social drama can all affect mental and emotional wellbeing, and since our hormones tend to snowball once stress kicks in, we can also see the physical effects of daily stress. While these are normal, everyday occurrences, you might be more sensitive to any stressors that take place during your fasting period.

While chronic stress can affect intermittent fasting in its entirety, a large dose of daily stress can make that period of fasting way more uncomfortable than it needs to be.

"Taking it slow" can be amazingly beneficial to reducing daily stress. If you wake up with 20 minutes to get to work or school, that leaves you scrambling to get up, get ready, and get out the door. And then there's the stress of actually making it there on time, and even more stress if you end up being late. While hitting the ground running can be a great strategy in many scenarios, it isn't the best way to start your day. It gets your adrenaline pumping, and when you're fasting, the repercussions of that (which include hunger) are probably not something you want to deal with.

When you're regulating your sleep schedule at the start of your fast, consider waking up earlier than you necessarily need to. Adding an extra hour or two prior to your daily responsibilities can be very healthy, mentally and physically. It allows you to take your time waking up and gives you more time to take care of yourself—which can be difficult to do if you're on a time crunch to get out the door.

Use this extra time to take a shower, catch up on your favorite show, read a book, do chores that you're behind on... whatever is satisfying or relaxing to you, and will make the rest of your day feel less rushed.

However, you've scheduled your eating/fasting periods, make sure that you can always consume something once your eating window begins. This is extremely important.

If you're stuck in traffic once 2PM rolls around, the knowledge that it's time to eat (right now, as your ghrelin levels will tell you) will make the agony of sitting in traffic even more exaggerated. It's definitely a good idea to carry snacks on you if your daily life is busy so that you have something to eat as soon as you're allowed to. Hardboiled eggs, nut and seed mixes, or fresh or dried fruit are always nice to have on hand. They've got the protein, glucose, and fats that your body will be desperately craving.

If you have time in the day to hit the gym, it's a good idea to also do this around the same time each day—specifically in correlation to your fast. If you begin exercising right before your first meal of the day, skipping this for too many days in a row can reduce the fat burning affects you see over time, and might make you feel more lethargic after eating. If you opt to exercise in the middle of your fast, it could have the regrettable side effect of triggering your hunger hormones way too early. It is okay to switch up your exercise routine occasionally—but consistency is important, especially while you're fasting. If it's hard for you to know when or how long to exercise, having a discussion with a personal trainer or fitness instructor to figure out a personalized

workout plan for your fast may be very
beneficial.

Winding Down

This is by far the easiest part of the day to control because you don't have to worry about planning and preparing for the day ahead—just relaxing enough to get a good nights' rest. However, when it comes to regulating sleep schedules, this is where a lot of people can accidentally mess up.

It might actually be easier for our internal alarm clocks to wake us up at the same time each morning than it is for us to remember a consistent bedtime.

Doing things in the evening is fine—nobody wants to be the friend who never goes out to dinner or has late-night outings with friends. But as with everything else, moderation is extremely important. If friends or family are blowing your phone up at 11PM, trying to get you to go out with them, take a moment to remind them they have probably eaten twice as much as you in the last 24 hours and therefore have a lot more energy to expend than you. If possible, try to engage in social activities during the day so that the call of night-life doesn't ruin your routines and fast.

While actually getting to sleep at the same time each night might be hard at first, physically being in bed around the same time can make the process easier. This is something that a lot of us probably remember being told as kids. If you're laying down, it's a lot easier for your body to relax and wind down. And hopefully, waking up around the same time each morning will also make adhering to a regular bedtime a bit easier.

Fasting Isn't for Everyone

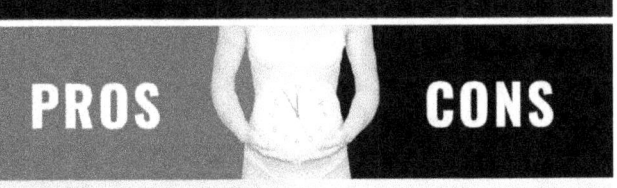

INTERMITTENT FASTING

PROS

- ✓ EASIER TO IMPLEMENT THAN TRADITIONAL DIETING
- ✓ HELPS SUPPRESS INFLAMMATION AND FIGHT FREE RADICAL DAMAGE
- ✓ GREAT WAY TO PRACTICE MANAGING HUNGER

CONS

- ⊗ RESEARCH SHOWS THAT IT'S NOT BETTER THAN TRADITIONAL CALORIC RESTRICTION
- ⊗ NOT GOOD FOR PEOPLE WITH POOR GLYCEMIC CONTROL
- ⊗ MAY LEAD TO BINGE EATING

Since intermittent fasting has such an impactful domino effect on our hormones and reproductive processes, there are certain cases in which it might be risky engaging in a fast—even for a few days. Among other factors, chronic stress, insomnia, or having a history of disordered eating are all things to consider when you're thinking about trying a new diet.

Fasting while pregnant can pose some severe risks and should not be attempted. When a female is pregnant, the fetus is absorbing a significant amount of the nutrients that would otherwise be going to the mother. Cutting meals and snacks can lead to a significant decline in health while pregnant. This is one of the reasons that ovulation and reproductive hormones may be negatively impacted at the start of a fast: your body knows that becoming pregnant during a time of famine or food shortage could be lethal. If you begin a fast while actively pregnant, your body doesn't have a chance to adjust to the potential risks of lower food intake and might compensate by sending all your nutrients to the fetus instead you.

Other factors such as insomnia or high levels of stress should also be taken into consideration before you begin a fast of any length. Lack of sleep or excessive stress are already stressors that your body is coping with and adding another stressor (like fasting) on top of that could be very detrimental to your overall health. If you don't sleep well, your hormones might already be out of whack, leading to mood swings, irregular ovulation in women, or trouble maintaining weight and muscle in men and women. The same can be said for chronic stress since it also plays directly off your hormones.

If you have concerns about your health history, you should always consult with your doctor before beginning any major dietary changes. After all, everyone's body and nutritional needs are unique, so what works exquisitely for some might have severely detrimental effects for others. There are always other methods of losing weight and improving overall health; it is important that you choose the path that's right for you.

Alternatives to Intermittent Fasting

If the time isn't right for you to try fasting, or if you're trying it and it just isn't working out, there are many other methods and diets you can try. The important part is making sure you're getting an adequate amount of nutrients and macronutrients, staying active, and maintaining an overall healthy lifestyle. Some popular plans that may help you see some of the core benefits of intermittently fasting are the ketogenic diet, whole food or paleo diets, and eating many small meals a day instead of three large ones - I wrote a book with recipes, which you can always find on Amazon, under this heading → Keto Meal Prep Cookbook: Beginners Ketogenic Diet For Weight Loss With Low-Carb Food.

Keto, Paleo, and whole food diets all have the same core principal: they exclude the foods that we don't absolutely need to survive, or rather, they consist mainly of foods that some of our most ancient ancestors may have eaten and thrived on. In all these diets, grains and sugars are strongly advised against. Keto excludes them because they inhibit your body's ability to run purely off ketones instead of glucose. Paleo cuts them out because in the Paleolithic era, our ancestors were hunters and gatherers with no access to farmed grains or processed foods, meaning they are not necessary to our survival and development. Simplest of all, whole food diets don't contain many refined grains or sugars because whole, natural foods just don't have them.

If you are looking for a diet that has strong backing from an evolutionary standpoint, any of these are worth exploring. They are malleable, but not to the point of being ineffective. Keto is by far the strictest regimen on the list since it has the most specific guidelines and goals.

With Paleo or whole foods, nearly any dietary restrictions—vegan, gluten free, lactose intolerant, nut allergies—are easily accommodated without missing out on a significant amount of variety.

And to their credit, all of these diets have been shown to reduce excess body fat, increase insulin sensitivity, and improve general health and wellness.

Conclusion

Thank you for making it to the end of Intermittent Fasting Plan: A Guide to Losing Weight. Care Your Body Through Lessons to Reset Diet, Motivational Habits & Delicious Recipes. Let's hope it was informative and able to provide you with all the tools needed to complete your goals whatever they may be. While this book aimed to be all-encompassing, intermittent fasting and other dietary plans are extremely complex, and always worth looking further into. It is very important that you choose whatever plan that best matches your personal needs.

The next step is to take a break from the books and evaluate your situation as it is right now. Why are you pursuing intermittent fasting? Are you aiming to lose weight, battling a chronic illness, and hoping for relief, or just want to generally increase your quality of life? Make sure you know where you stand before leaping into anything; your health depends on it.

If you plan on moving forward with intermittent fasting, then congratulations and good luck! You should set aside some time to get a game plan together. Stockpile your favorite coffee, teas, and electrolyte supplements to make the transition easier. If you want to try fasting in tandem with another diet, make sure you have a variety of foods that will meet your nutritional needs as well as your dietary ones.

Have a few extra layers ready for when the fasting coldness hits and some extra water bottles on hand.

Mentally buckle up for some wicked hunger pangs but know that they won't last long. Tell your friends and family about your diet plan—have them hold you to it and help you along the way. And remember: the first few days will be rough, but you've got this. Whether your goal is weight loss or wellbeing, you've taken the first step by learning, and now you're ready to hit the ground running.

--- eBook 2 ---

KETO MEAL

PREP

COOKBOOK

Beginners Ketogenic Diet

For Weight Loss

With Low-Carb Food

Introduction

Congratulations for purchasing **Keto Meal Prep Cookbook**: <u>Beginner Ketogenic Diet For Weight Loss With Low-Carb Food</u> and thank you for doing so.

I believe the information provided will give you a jump start to enjoying an array of delicious meals and snacks to switch your body into a state of ketosis. You can enjoy a healthier and yet delicious meal and snack options.

The following chapters will discuss how to cook your meals as you try to shuffle a hectic schedule to prepare tasty items for your family. You will discover how important planning is when it's time to visit the grocery store. The only way is to plan ahead of time and purchase all of the essential items and store them until needed. You will be provided with a 21-Day meal plan to get yourself off to the right start.

Keep your prep going because you'll get spoiled how simple it is to maintain a healthy diet and subsequently, a healthy lifestyle. The plan will work whether you are prepping for two days or a week. Choose a day when you don't have any pressing obligations, get tossing and bake or plan the meals you want to prepare for your family.

I believe that you will enjoy each segment of Keto Meal Prep Cookbook: Beginner Ketogenic Diet For Weight-Loss With Low-Carb Food since it is catered to your satisfactory life-changing habits. The recipes are carefully selected with the lowest possible carbs as you prepare each of your meals. The meal plan is sufficient to get you started. If you have a preference or don't enjoy the items as they are listed on the menu, merely swap it out for one of the others you will enjoy. Every recipe provided has the balanced carbohydrates, protein, and total fats listed for your convenience.

Please enjoy !

Chapter 1

<u>Fundamentals of the</u>
<u>Ketogenic Diet</u>

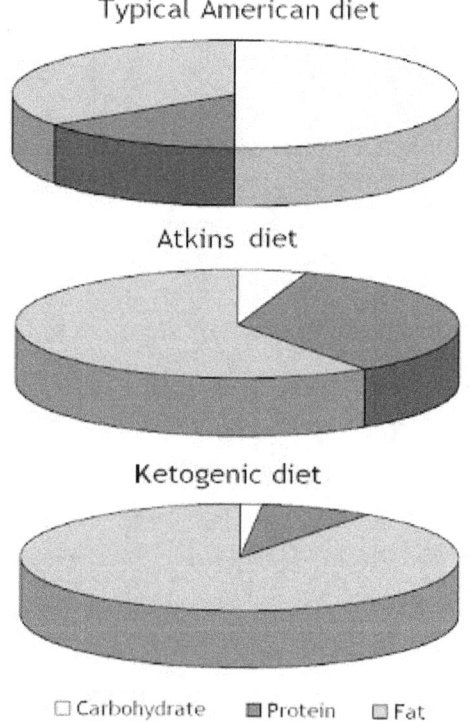

Typical American diet

Atkins diet

Ketogenic diet

☐ Carbohydrate ■ Protein ☐ Fat

You may feel a bit challenged as you begin your new way of dieting, but it will be so worth it. The ketogenic methods described will work best if combined with a bit of light exercise. With the right balance of carbs, fats, and proteins, you will be on the way to ketosis. Ketosis is used to help you drop extra pounds and burn body fat using healthy eating practices. Proteins will fuel your body to burn the fat, which in turn, ketosis will maintain your muscles and make you less hungry.

Your body will remain healthy and work as it should. If you don't consume enough carbs from your food, your cells will begin to burn fat for the necessary energy instead. Your body will switch over to ketosis for its energy source as you cut back on your calories and carbs.

Two events occur when your body doesn't need the glucose. The first stage involves glycogenesis which is where the excess of glucose will convert to glycogen which is stored in the liver and your muscles. Research indicates that only about half of your energy used daily can be saved as glycogen. The second stage is lipogenesis. If your body does not receive that supply of glycogen for your muscles and liver, then it is converted to fat and stored.

The ketogenesis process begins once the glycerol and fatty acid molecules are released and acetoacetate is produced. The acetoacetate is converted to two specific types of ketone elements. The first type is the acetone which is mainly excreted as waste but can also become metabolized into glucose which causes the foul-smelling breath when you reach ketosis. Beta-hydroxybutyrate/BHB is also produced whereas your muscles will convert the acetoacetate into BHB which fuels your brain after you have been on the keto diet for a short time.

Your body will have no more food (similar to when you are sleeping) making your body burn the fat to create ketones. Once the ketones break down the fats which generate fatty acids, they will burn-off in the liver through beta-oxidation. Thus, when you no longer have a supply of glycogen or glucose, ketosis begins and will use the consumed/stored fat as energy.

Types of Keto Diets

The Standard Ketogenic Diet or the SKD Plan: Typically, this diet is a low- carbohydrate (5% average), high-fat (75% average), and moderate protein (20%) diet plan. Note: These are average counts and can vary.

The Targeted Ketogenic Diet or the TKD Plan: This is the one you need when you are training or working out. You can add more carbs around your workouts and still remain in ketosis.

The High-Protein Ketogenic Diet: This plan is comparable to the SKD plan but consists of more protein. Its ratio is repeatedly noted as maintaining 35% protein, 5% carbs, and 60% fat. (Once again, these are average percentages.)

The Cyclical Ketogenic Diet or the CKD Plan:

This particular plan generally has five regular ketogenic days with two days of high-carbohydrates to follow (the 5:2 technique). The program involves higher carbohydrate refeeds, meaning it is a predetermined time of higher carb/calorie overfeeding during a caloric deficit.

How Long it Takes to Get into Ketosis

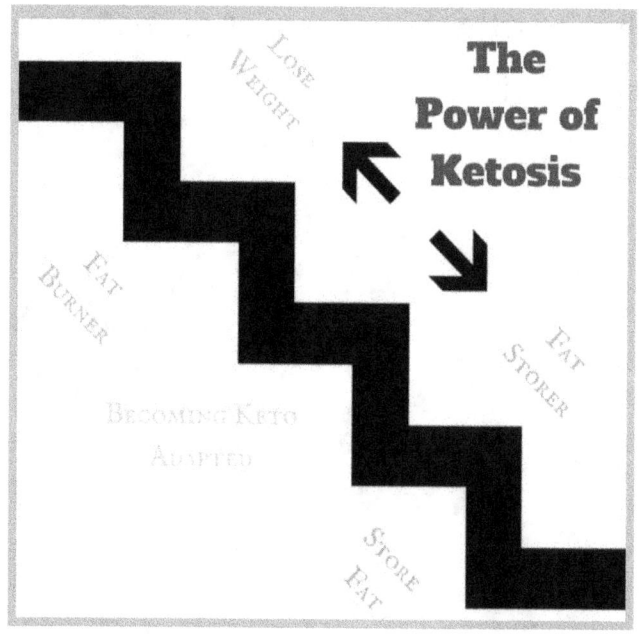

As you focus on weight loss, you have to realize each person will enter ketosis at a different rate. If you remain under your optimal net carb limits, you should reach it within two to three days. However, since human research is limited, most studies indicate most techniques chosen rarely take more than two weeks. Many have reached ketosis within one week.

Exercise on an empty stomach is the fastest method you can use since it will accelerate the depletion of your body's glycogen. Try a Fat Fast for 2-3 days where you consume more fat to speed up your ketosis rate. Remove all of the refined carbs including sugar. You can also do a water fast where you just drink water to speed up the pace of ketosis.

Carbohydrate Intake Monitored

Ideally, you want to take in less than 50 grams each day (20 is ideal). So that you realize how high carbs can range, check out these totals:

- Oatmeal – 1/2 cup – 12 grams
- Strawberries – 1 cup – 11 grams
- Almonds – 3/4 of 1 cup – 26-30 carbs
- Banana – 1 medium – 27 carbs
- Chocolate Milk – 1 cup – 26-30 carbs
- Sweet Potatoes – 28 carbs – 1 cup
- Peas or Corn – 1/2 cup – 15 gram

Even in small portions, foods you eat in your typical diet plan can add up fast. Consider these classifications in your ketogenic diet →

If you choose moderate intake of carbs: Consume 100-150 grams of carbohydrates each day if you are lean and active or are making an attempt to maintain a specific weight. Enjoy all of the veggies you desire, have several fruit portions and a few healthy starches including, oats, rice, potatoes, or sweet potatoes.

If you take the medium carb route: Consume 50-100 grams each day by enjoying two to three pieces of fruit, a ton of vegetables, and minimal starchy carbohydrates.

If you choose the high road to maximize weight loss: Since you will be using the intermittent fasting times, you will probably want to use the ratios of 20-50 grams of carbs each day. This allotment is particularly essential for those who suffer from diabetes, are metabolically deranged, or are obese. Your body will achieve the state of ketosis which supplies the ketone bodies.

Balance Your Eating Habits

Exercise is a significant element to the success of the ketogenic diet plan. Cortisol is a hormone which is released from your adrenal gland in response to chemical signs or other stress signals. You should consider exercising 30-60 minutes daily as an integral part of healthy living choices.

Regular physical activity benefits your strength, mood, and balance. If you've been living a more sedentary lifestyle, it's vital for you to speak with your doctor about a safe exercise regimen. Make sure you start off slow. Progressively 'pick up the pace' and regularity of your workouts.

Choose Protein to Make the Balance for Weight Loss

It's vital to maintain and preserve your calorie-burning lean muscles. Your body cannot use and burn your fat intake unless you provide either protein or carbohydrates. Your digestion process is slowed which in turn makes you satisfied with the foods you consume using the ketogenic techniques. You want to remove all of the temptations to eliminate cheating. By consuming fruits and veggies with the low-carbs, you are reducing many of those unwanted calories.

It is best to increase your carbohydrate intake on days you are more active, such as training or working out times. You need to balance the calories, carbs, and proteins to achieve your weight loss goals. The keto diet is perfect for this important focus.

Achieving Ketosis

You may be unsure if you have reached your ketogenic status. You will be plagued with several body functions including the following symptoms →

Nasty Breath: You may notice a metallic or fruity taste with an odor similar to nail polish remover. This is the by-product of acetoacetic acid (acetone) which is a visible indication. You may also experience a drier mouth. These changes are normal as a side effect as your body processes these high-fat foods. Once you are accustomed to the ketogenic dieting techniques, the lousy breath symptoms will pass. If you are socializing, try a diet soda or a no-sugar drink. Sugar-free gum is also a quick fix. Always check the nutrition labels for carbohydrate facts, you may be surprised. These are not allowed on the keto diet because they reduce ketones. Therefore, only use it temporarily. If you are at home, just grab the toothbrush.

Changes in Your Sleep Patterns: After you have a good night of sleep, your body is in ketosis since you have fasted for over eight hours, you are on the way to burning ketones. If you are new to the high-fat and low-carb dieting, the optimal fat-burning state takes time. Your body has depended on bringing in carbs and glucose, it will not readily give up carbs and start to crave saturated fats.

The restless night is also a normal side effect. Vitamin supplements can sometimes remedy the problem that can be caused by a lowered insulin and serotonin level. For a quick fix, try one-half of a tablespoon of fruit spread and a square of chocolate.

Smelly Urine: With the high acetone levels, your urine is also a strong clue to ketosis. There's no reason for concern, it's merely your body adjusting to the new status.

Reduced Appetite: When you reduce your carbs and proteins, you will be increasing your fat intake. The decreased appetite comes from the multitude of fibrous veggies, fats, and satiating nutrients provided in the new diet.

The 'full' factor is a huge benefit to the ketogenic plan. It will give you one less thing to worry about – being hungry.

<u>Benefits of the Keto Diet</u>

Does Keto Burn more fat ?

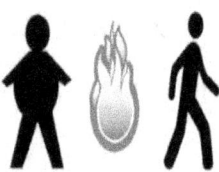

Will You Get Keto Flu ?   Is It A Low Carb

High Protein Diet ?

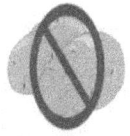

Does Keto Boost Metabolism ?

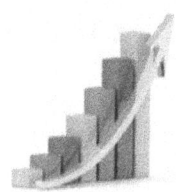

As you begin your new ketogenic way of life, you must understand that no two people will have the same benefits. You will be living a much healthier way of living which will include many benefits. These are just a few of the ways which keto will get your life into balance.

Receive increase of energy: This happens as your body breaks down the fats instead of carbs. Think of the balance using the energy content of nutrients.

Achieve fewer seizure episodes for epilepsy individuals: The therapeutic keto diet used for epilepsy can restrict the carb intake daily to less than 15 grams which significantly increases the ketone levels. Please understand that you should not attempt these low ratios unless you are supervised by a professional dietitian or another medical official.

Cognitive performance will improve: In ketosis, you have a reduction of glucose, your brain will begin to use ketones as fuel resulting in a decrease in the level of toxins. Therefore, your concentration and productivity will improve.

Provides relief for those who suffer from mild Alzheimer's disease: You first need to realize the human brain is an energy hog and demands a constant supply of fuel. However, those suffering from Dementia have difficulty burning blood sugar or glucose. That deficiency can lead to 'sluggish' brain activity. Luckily, except in advanced cases, the brain has no problem burning the ketones for fuel which is provided by the low-carb keto diet plan.

Cholesterol profile will be improved: An arterial buildup is generally associated with the triglyceride and cholesterol levels. Many have been reported to have upgrading results with the use of the keto diet techniques.

Drastic drops in the levels of triglycerides are possible: The triglycerides are the fat molecules that are present in your bloodstream. High levels can place you at high-risk factor for heart disease. Carb consumption is the primary driver of those elevated levels.

Improvement for Pre-Diabetes & Diabetes individuals: By removing the excess of fat by using the ketogenic plan, you are also improving your insulin sensitivity, lowering inflammation, and directly reducing your blood sugar. Since ketones are fuel and a metabolic regulator, it makes nutritional ketosis a very suitable option for reversing type 2 Diabetes.

Lower blood pressure is a plus: A low-carb diet plan can help lower your pressure. You may also need to decrease any medications you are currently taking, so be sure you ask your physician before you begin. Thus, one of the symptoms that ketosis is working will be recognized with a lower pressure rate.

Cancer can improve: According to lab research, keto supplementation can decrease the tumor cell viability and prolong the survival of mice with metastatic cancer.

Polycystic Ovary Syndrome (PCOS) improvements: This is the utmost endocrine disorder affecting young women of child-bearing years and is also associated with insulin resistance, obesity, and hyperinsulinemia. A six-month study concluded a significant improvement in weight with fasting women over a 24-week period. The group limited carb intake to 20 grams daily for the 24 weeks' time period.

Dental hygiene improves: If you are prone to tooth decay or gum disease, you will be glad to know keto can help. The balance of pH in your mouth is influenced by the intake of sugar. Since the keto techniques used are lower in sugar, you should have improvement of ongoing issues after about three months. You will be eating healthier fruits and not sugary snacks or desserts.

Natural weight loss: The balanced meals featuring high fats and low carbohydrates help remove those unwanted inches around your waistline. As you lower the carb intake in your body, you will also be increasing the fats included in the keto diet. The multitude of fats, fiber-filled veggies, and satiating nutrients provided in the new diet plan will boost the 'full' factor, making this a significant benefit to the ketogenic plan.

Metabolic Syndrome patients have relief: This is associated with your risk of heart disease and diabetes. It carries its own symptoms including low HDL cholesterol levels, elevated blood pressure, high triglycerides, elevated fasting blood sugar levels, and abdominal obesity. The low-carb diet plan helps with these issues and many are nearly eliminated.

A special note for women: Somewhere along the path, women began to believe that fat was bad and caused weight gain. You now realize this is a myth! You are gaining new methods to improve your health and so much more using the low carb and high-fat techniques combined in keto. Just recall, these are some of your unique advantages using the ketogenic methods if you have any of these symptoms:

- You want to increase your workout performance in the gym
- Have adrenal fatigue
- Feel tired or unmotivated
- Have PCOS
- Have terrible PMS
- Have irregular or absent periods
- Have imbalanced thyroid hormones
- Cannot lose or gain weight no matter what you try
- Get hungry and need to always have a snack handy in between meals
- Have an autoimmune disease you would like to manage

Get Started With Essential Tools

Each of these tools will help you speed up the cooking needs while preparing your keto meals.

Purchase a good set of weighing scales: You can take out the guesswork with a set of scales. The scale should have a tare function so when you set a bowl on the scale, the feature will allow you to reset the range back to zero. Also, seek one with a conversion button. You need to know how to convert measurements into grams since not all recipes have them listed. The grams keep the system in line. Keep the germs off of the scale by removing the plate. Be sure it's removable to eliminate the bacterial buildup.

Take advantage of your instant pot, crockpot, & slow cooker: You will find the crockpot a must if you have a busy lifestyle. These are just a couple of ways you can benefit from its use:

- Save a ton of effort and time: All it takes is a few good recipes and a little bit of your valuable time. In most of the cases, these recipes are geared towards a fast lifestyle and will be ready with just a few simple steps. After some time and practice, you will know which ones will be your favorites.

- Get ahead of the meal: Preparing food with your slow cooker can put you ahead of the game. You can prepare the cooker the night before if you have a busy day planned. All it takes is a few minutes of preparation. Just add all of the fixings into the pot and place it in the fridge - overnight. The next morning, transfer to the counter to become room temperature. Turn it on as you head out of the door and your meal or dessert will be ready when you get home.

Purchase a food processor, immersion blender or regular blender: Each of these will be an essential part of preparing many of the recipes for your special meals, desserts, and snacks.

Purchase accurate measuring tools: A measuring cup and spoon system that shows both the Metric and US standards of weight is essential, so there is no confusion during prep.

Buy a spiralizer or a sharp knife: You can prepare 'zoodles' which are noodles cut from zucchini easily.

Chapter 2

Ketogenic Diet Do's & Don'ts

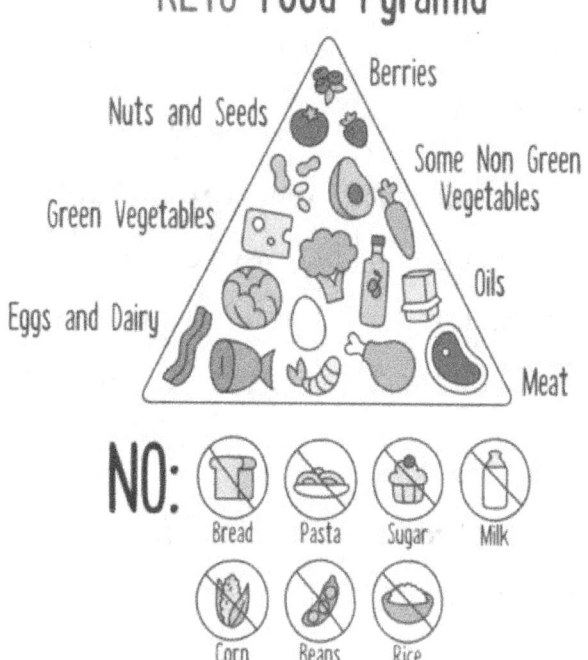

Transitioning into the ketogenic way of living can be made easier by using low-carb substitutions for common goods used in cooking and baking. These are just a few ways keto-friendly products can be used to save the carbohydrates and provide you with an alternative plan. We will work starting with the pantry stock including flour, sweeteners, spices, and other products you will need to help keep your carbs under control while you are dropping the pounds. Also, you will learn in depth which veggies and fruits are suitable for your ketogenic plan.

Let's begin!

Flours and Thickening Substitutions →

- **Almond flour:** Almond flour is a suitable replacement and is used as all-purpose flour. Each one-quarter cup portion is only 3 carbohydrates per gram. The process involves blanching the almonds in boiling water to remove the skins. Next, you will grind the flour into a finely ground product that is an excellent choice for cakes, cookies, and pie crusts.

- **Almond meal:** Almond meal isn't identical to almond flour. However, it is still a good substitute if you're out of almond flour for baked goods. The only difference is that the meal can be blanched (with the skins removed) or un-blanched. Its consistency is a coarser grind product.

- **Coconut flour:** You can use coconut flour in many of the keto diet meals. Here is the rundown:
  - When using coconut flour, remember it isn't a 1:1 ratio. In comparison, you can substitute as little as 1/3 cup to 1/4 cup of coconut flour.
  - Use one-part water to one-part coconut flour and whisk together to use as a thickening agent. Just add it to hot liquids such as soup.
  - It's high in fiber - making it super absorbent. You can add oils, eggs, and other liquids as needed.
  - Use the coconut flour at times you are sauteing or frying foods.

- **Flax meal:** Meal is versatile as an egg substitute as well as flour, but it does absorb lots of liquid.

- **Egg white protein powder:** Try adding the protein powder to provide more elasticity of gluten when you are making bread. The powder will also add more protein to your diet counts.

- **Whole psyllium husk:** Use the entire husk in doughs where you require more "stretchiness" such as what you would have in wheat flour. It's excellent for pizza dough, tortillas, or bread.

- **Psyllium husk powder:** Fiber is its main ingredient, but it is combined with other low-carb flowers. You will need to add plenty of liquids to your baking items such as muffins or bread.

- **Sesame flour:** Finely grind sesame seeds to prepare the flour into the texture similar to wheat flour. Combine with psyllium flour for your baking needs to ensure the light texture of high-carb white bread.

Healthy Spices to the Rescue

As you begin gearing up for the keto-friendly kitchen, you will discover there are many spices you can prepare in the convenience of your home and have full knowledge of its components. Most of the spices listed are used frequently and have health benefits as well. Let's get stocking.

Purchase high-quality salts: Your insulin levels will decrease while you are engaging the ketogenic lifestyle. Higher sodium levels are naturally expelled by your kidneys. As a result, they lower the potassium/sodium ratio in your body. You can increase the amount of sodium with one of these choices:

- Add 1/4 teaspoon of pink salt to your food or into a glass of water.
- Eat a snack of pumpkin seeds or macadamia nuts.
- Enjoy a bowl of bone broth or use it in a keto recipe.
- Add kelp or nori to your prepared foods.
- Slice celery and cucumber – both have natural sodium content.

Prepare foods using cumin spice: Cumin is considered an antioxidant and as an excellent digestion reliever. It is a superior method to treat disorders such as asthma and bronchitis. It is also a great spice if you suffer from Diabetes or Prediabetics. It provides your body with iron, vitamins A & C, as well as being an excellent choice to assist in the removal of body fat.

Warm it up with cayenne pepper hot spices: Your metabolism will be increased to help burn away the fat since cayenne is actually a stimulant for digestive enzymes which also helps prevent stomach ulcers. Its anti-inflammatory elements make it a super choice for headaches, arthritis, or sore muscles. You can also receive a boost in your immunity as it clears away nasal congestion. Sprinkle your meatloaf, chili, soups, stews, or even your morning eggs.

Select basil as an anti-inflammatory herb: You can use fresh or dried basil to maximize its benefits. Its dark green color is an indication it also maintains an outstanding source of magnesium, calcium, and vitamin K which is excellent for your bones. These are some of the conditions it helps:

- Arthritis
- Allergies
- Inflammatory bowel conditions

Grind ground chia seeds: The seeds can absorb up to 11 times its weight in liquid. Be sure to add plenty of water and soak them for at least 5 minutes before using in your keto recipes. Otherwise, you will have some uncomfortable digestion after eating them. Be sure to remain hydrated.

Use star anise: This is one spice that is commonly used in Indian, Chinese, Indonesian, and Malaysian dishes. Its licorice-like taste pairs with tomatoes. It can be found as a 'star' as a whole piece or as a powder form. You can substitute for Chinese Five

Spice, common anise, or fennel seed. It is a super choice for its antifungal, antibacterial, and antioxidant qualities.

Turmeric spices to jazz it up: Dating back to Ayurveda and Chinese medicine - this Asian orange herb has been known for its anti-inflammatory elements. It is so easy to add to your delicious meats, veggies, and smoothies. These are some of its benefits:

- Excellent for weight management
- Relieves arthritis
- Helps Prevent Alzheimer's disease
- Improves your digestion
- Reduces your cholesterol levels
- Helps control diabetes

Prep A Batch Of Poultry Seasoning:

What you need:

- Dried sage – 2 tbsp.
- Dried marjoram – 1 tbsp.
- Ground nutmeg- .5 tbsp.
- Dried rosemary - .5 tbsp.
- Dried thyme – 1.5 tbsp.
- Ground black pepper - .5 tbsp.

How to prepare:

1. Mix each of the spices in a small jar or another type of storage container.
2. Use freely any time you want a little kick to your poultry.

Make your homemade pumpkin pie spice: Use this simple low-carb concoction and you know it will be healthy.

Yields: 10.75 tsp. @ 1 tsp. per serving

Macros: 0.8 g Net Carbs | 6.42 Calories | 0.12 g Protein |0.09 g Total Fats

What you need:

- Ground cinnamon – 2 tbsp.
- Ground nutmeg - .5 tsp.
- Ground ginger – 1 tbsp.
- Allspice - .5 tsp
- Cardamom - .25 tsp.
- Ground cloves - .5 tsp. or .75 tsp. whole cloves

How to prepare:

1. Use a spice grinder to grind the cloves into powder.
2. Combine all of the components into a large mixing container until combined thoroughly.
3. Store in a spice container to use any time the need arises.

Use sweet & spicy cloves: Add cloves to hot tea for a spicy flavor. The antiseptic and germicidal ingredients in cloves will help with many types of pain including:

- Helps relieve arthritis pain
- Helps relieve gum and tooth pain
- Relief of digestive problems
- Fights infections
- The smell of cloves can help encourage mental creativity

Oil of clove is beneficial as an antiseptic to kill bacteria in fungal infections, itchy rashes, bruises, or burns.

Apple cider vinegar: You can add just one to two tablespoons of vinegar to an 8-ounce glass of water to help the process or just take a shot of vinegar solo. These are just a few ways this helps your progress:

- Helps you to drop the pounds
- Helps with sore muscles
- Improves your digestion tract
- Excellent for detoxification
- A good energy booster
- Reduces cholesterol
- Controls sugar intake/aids in diabetes
- Strengthens your immune system
- Balances your inner body system and functions

Food Item Substitutions

Breadcrumbs substitution: Enjoy the same crunchy menu items by substituting regular breadcrumbs with crushed pork rinds. The healthier option offers zero carbs.

Replace the regular rice & potatoes: Exchange the regular serving portions of white or brown with cauliflower rice which is a much healthier option. You can also serve them for variety as mashed potatoes.

Try a pasta substitute: Replace pasta using zucchini. You use a spiralizer or sharp knife and make long ribbons to cover your plate. It is excellent for many dishes served this way. Think of how attractive it will be with a keto-friendly sauce.

Exchange your tortilla: Enjoy a leaf of lettuce for about one gram per serving and keep the healthy crunch.

Nuts & Seeds: You can choose from an array of nuts in moderation.

The number of carbs represents the net carbs which equal approximately 3.5 ounces:

- Chia Seeds – 0 grams
- Flax seeds – 0 grams
- Brazil nuts – 4 grams
- Pecans – 4 grams
- Macadamia – 5 grams
- Hazelnuts – 7 grams
- Peanuts – 7 grams
- Walnuts – 7 grams
- Peanuts – 7 grams
- Pine nuts – 9 grams
- Almonds – 10 grams
- Pumpkin seeds – 14.3 grams

- Sesame seeds – 17.7 grams
- Pistachios – 18 grams

In comparison, you now see why those potato chips are 48 grams and M&Ms are 70 grams.

Choose fermented foods & probiotics: Enjoy a dish of yogurt. You can also include items such as kimchee, sauerkraut, pickles, coconut milk or water kefir to benefit your digestive system. Fermented foods help restore the 'good' bacteria in your gut. The natural acids help stabilize your blood sugar levels as well as the enzymes, probiotics, and other bioactive nutrients help support ketosis.

Add plenty of limes & lemons to your diet plan: Your blood sugar levels will naturally drop with these citric additions and signal a boost in your liver function. Use them with a salad, in green juices, or with cooked with meats or veggies. The choices are limitless and assist you with the following:

- Boosts your immune system
- Excellent for weight loss
- Balances pH
- Relieves respiratory infections
- Reduces fever
- Blood purifier
- Reduces toothache pain
- Decreases wrinkles and blemishes
- Flushes out the unwanted, unhealthy materials

Choose Healthy Fats & Oils

Use coconut oil: You vamp up the fat intake with this high flash-point oil. Enjoy a coconut oil smoothie before your workouts. Use it with your meats, chicken, fish, or on top of veggies. It will quickly transfer from solid form to oil according to its temperature.

Add extra-virgin olive oil (EVOO): Olive oil dates back for centuries – back to where oil was used for anointing kings and priests. High-quality oil with its low-acidity makes the EVOO have a smoke point as high as 410ºF. That's higher than most cooking applications call for, making olive oil more heat-stable than many other cooking fats. It contains (2 tsp.) - 0 carbs.

Monounsaturated fats, such as the ones in olive oil, are also linked with better blood sugar regulation, including lower fasting glucose, as well as reducing inflammation throughout the body. Olive oil also helps to prevent cardiovascular disease by protecting the integrity of your vascular system and lowering LDL which is also called the 'bad' cholesterol.

Add macadamia oil: One of the benefits of this oil is that it has a high smoke point. It carries a mild flavor which is a super alternative to olive oil in mayonnaise.

Other monounsaturated and saturated fats: Include these items (listed in grams):

- Olives – 3 jumbo - 5 large or 10 small – 1 gram of net carbs
- Avocado oil – 1 tbsp. – 0 net carbs
- Chicken fat – 1 tbsp. – 0 net carbs
- Duck Fat – 1 tbsp. – 0 net carbs
- Beef Tallow – 1 tbsp. – 0 net carbs
- Unsweetened flaked coconut – 3 tbsp. – 2 net carbs
- Unsalted Butter – 1 tbsp. – 0 net carbs
- Ghee - 1 tsp. – 0 net carbs
- Egg yolks – 1 large – 0.6 net carbs
- Organic Red Palm oil – ex. Nutivia - 1 tbsp. – 0 net carbs
- Sesame oil – 1 tbsp. – 0 net carbs
- Flaxseed oil – 1 tbsp. – 0 net carbs
- Various dressings – see recipes
- Keto-friendly mayonnaise – see recipes

Choose Healthy Protein Options

It is recommended to use grass-fed, organic, pasture-raised meats when they are available. Provide these for your baking and cooking needs while dieting with keto and fasting.

- Eggs
- Fresh Seeds & Nuts: Chia seeds, sesame seeds, flax seeds, macadamia nuts are excellent choices.
- Turkey breasts & ground turkey
- Chicken breasts, ground chicken, thighs, and drumsticks
- Other Poultry: Pheasant & Quail
- Shrimp, lobster, crawfish, squid, octopus, crab, or oysters
- Sardines
- Fresh or canned tuna
- Fresh wild-caught salmon
- Pork chops

- Beef: Chuck roast, lean ground beef, flank steak, sirloin, etc.
- Venison is a delicious lean choice
- Cured Meats: Prosciutto, salami, or pepperoni

Always Have Fresh Fruit Handy

You can enjoy 1/2 of a cup of each of these items:

- Apples – no skin – boiled – 13.6 grams
- Apricots – 7.5 grams
- Bananas – 23.4 grams
- Blackberries – 23 grams
- Blueberries – 22 grams
- Cantaloupe – 6 grams
- Kiwi – 14.2 grams
- Oranges – 12 grams
- Peaches – 12 grams
- Pears – 19.2 grams
- Pineapple – 11 grams
- Plums – 16.3 grams
- Kiwi – 15 grams
- Watermelon – 7.1 grams

These are few more fruits that are acceptable for the Keto diet plan:

- Avocados
- Coconut
- Lemon juice
- Lime juice
- Strawberries
- Casaba Melon
- Green olives
- Rhubarb
- Black Olive
- Oheloberries
- Boysenberries
- Grapefruit
- Carambola aka Starfruit
- Gooseberries
- Acerola - aka West Indian Cherry

Choose Keto-Friendly Sweeteners

Xylitol is at the top of the sugary list as an excellent choice to sweeten your teriyaki and barbecue sauce and teriyaki. Its natural-occurring sugar alcohol has a Glycemic index (GI) standing of 13. Xylitol also helps keep your mouth bacteria in check and is commonly found in chewing gum. However, don't use it often in large amounts since it can cause diarrhea, making chewing gum a laxative if used in large quantities. Note: It is toxic for dogs even in small amounts.

Stevia drops offer delicious flavors including hazelnut, vanilla, English toffee, and chocolate. Enjoy making a satisfying cup of sweetened coffee or other healthy drinks. Some individuals think the drops are too bitter, so at first, use only three drops to equal one teaspoon of sugar.

Pyure's organic all-purpose blend is well-thought-out the best all-around sweetener with less of a bitter after-taste versus a stevia-based product. The blend of stevia and erythritol is an excellent alternative to baking, sweetening desserts, and various cooking needs. The substitution ratio is one teaspoon of sugar for each one-third teaspoon of Pyure. Just add the blend slowly and adjust to your taste. If you need powdered sugar, just grind the sweetener in a NutriBullet or high-speed blender until it maintains a dry consistency.

Swerve granular sweetener is also an excellent choice as a blend. It's made from non-digestible carbs sourced from starchy root veggies and select fruits. Start with 3/4 of a teaspoon for every one of sugar. Increase the portion to your taste.

Swerve confectioner's powdered sugar for your baking needs. Unfortunately, it's more expensive (about twice the price) than other products such as the Pyure.

For a brown sugar option: Golden Monk Fruit Sweetener is an excellent choice for brown sugar. The name monk-fruit came from the Buddhist monks over 1,000 years ago and is considered a cooling agent. It may not agree with your digestive system. Therefore, it's advisable to use it frugally if using in baked goods.

Pancake syrup: Lakanto's Maple-Flavored Syrup is an exceptional choice for pancake syrup since it is monk-fruit and erythritol based.

Understand the Glycemic Index (GI)

Each of these products has a GI next to them which measurement of how much your blood sugar is raised after you consume a specific food. If there is a zero (0) next to it, that means it will not increase your blood sugar counts. The measurement can reach 100 which is the baseline of insulin.

- Aspartame – GI: 0
- Erythritol – GI: 0
- Stevia (liquid) – GI: 0
- Monk Fruit – GI: 0
- Inulin – GI: 0
- Saccharin – GI: Variable
- Sucralose (liquid) GI: Variable
- Xylitol – GI: 13
- Maltitol – GI: 36

Stock the Refrigerator

- Grass-Fed Butter: You can promote fat loss and butter is almost carb-free. The butter is a naturally occurring fatty acid which is rich in conjugated linoleic acid (CLA). It is suitable for maintaining weight loss and retaining lean muscle mass.

- Ghee is also a great staple for your keto stock which is also called clarified butter.

- Whole eggs: Choose from Omega-3 eggs, whole eggs, and pasteurized eggs. Visit your local area market for free-range options. You can scramble, fry, boil, or devil eggs up for a picnic or any occasion for a quick snack.

- Heavy whipping cream: This is an option almost unbelievable with only 5 grams of fat per tablespoon.
- Kefir: Health benefits include supporting detoxification, building your bone density, fighting off some types of cancer, and many other issues.

Stock these items in the fridge for various recipes:

- Full-fat sour cream
- Goat cheese
- Full-fat cream cheese
- Parmesan cheese
- Hard & Soft cheeses – ex. mozzarella or sharp cheddar

If you're trying to lose weight and have hit a plateau, maybe you should limit your dairy intake. If you have a bloated feeling, you may also need a break from the heavy whipping cream and cheese.

Make Wise Beverages Choices

Stay hydrated and keep it simple by drinking tons of water to remain hydrated. Mayo Clinic concludes that men should drink about 15.5 cups of fluids daily and 11.5 cups for women. Consider some of these beverage choices. This chart is calculated with your grams of carbs derived for you:

- Water: 0 grams
- Water with lemon: 0 grams
- Plain Tea: 0 g – Note: You can add 1 sugar cube for 4 grams
- Plain Coffee: 0- grams
- 1 cup soy milk: 12 grams
- 1 cup coconut water: 9 grams

- 8 oz. almond milk: unsweetened - 2 grams
- 1 cup orange juice: 26 grams

Fresh or Frozen Vegetables

Each of these veggies is calculated for 1/2 cup servings:

- Alfalfa Seeds – Sprouted – 0.2 grams
- Arugula – 2.05 grams
- Asparagus – 1.78 grams
- Bamboo shoots – 3 grams
- Beans – Green snap – 3.6 grams
- Beet greens – 0.63 grams
- Broccoli – 4.04 grams
- Cabbage – Savoy – 3 grams
- Carrots – 6.8 grams
- Carrots – baby – 5.34 grams
- Cauliflower – 3 grams
- Celery – 1.4 grams
- Chard – 2 grams
- Chicory greens – 0.7 grams
- Chives – 1.9 grams

- Coriander – Cilantro Leaves – 0.87 grams
- Cucumber with Peel – 3.1 grams
- Eggplant – 2.9 grams
- Garlic – 33 grams
- Ginger root – 16 grams
- Kale – heart healthy with folate & magnesium – 5.2 grams
- Leeks – bulb (+) lower leaf – 12.4 grams
- Lemongrass – citronella – 25 grams
- Lettuce – red leaf – 1.4 grams
- Lettuce – crisp-head types ex. iceberg – 1.8 grams
- Mushrooms brown – 3.7 grams
- Mustard Greens – 1.5 grams
- Onions – yellow – 7.6 grams
- Onions – scallions or spring – 4.7 grams
- Onions – sweet – 6.7 grams
- Peppers – banana – 1.95 grams
- Peppers – jalapeno – 3.7 grams

- Peppers – red hot chili – 7.3 grams
- Peppers – sweet – green – 3 grams
- Peppers – sweet – red – 3.9 grams
- Peppers – sweet – yellow – 5.4 grams
- Portabella Mushrooms – 2.6 grams
- Pumpkin – 6 grams
- Radishes – 1.8 grams
- Seaweed – kelp – 8.3 grams
- Seaweed – spirulina – 2 grams
- Shiitake mushrooms – 4.3 grams
- Spinach – 1.4 grams
- Squash – crookneck – summer – 2.6 grams
- Squash - Zucchini – 2 grams
- Squash – winter – acorn – 8.9 grams
- Tomatoes – 2 grams
- Turnips – 4.6 grams
- Turnip Greens – 3.9 grams
- White Mushrooms – 2.3 grams

These veggies are also acceptable: Peas, squash, parsnips, and zucchini.

Foods You Should Not Eat

Hydrogenated fats: You need to avoid cold-pressed items when using vegetable oils which include safflower or soybean. This category also includes the use of margarine.

Avoid juices: You will get a burst of energy from the juice but just a 12 oz. portion of unsweetened apple juice packs 48 grams of carbohydrates. The delicious unsweetened grape juice passes that one for a 12 oz. serving - weighing in at 60 grams per serving – only 2 carbs from the fiber. Keep in mind, that drinking juice can lead to hunger pangs and more unplanned snacking. It's probably easier to avoid it when possible.

Regular dairy milk: You can avoid the extra carbs by using a non-dairy option.

Avoid these fruits: Consume these in small portions due to high-carb content: cranberries, blueberries, raspberries, and strawberries.

Avoid starchy veggies: You need to avoid large amounts of beans and legumes. Even though they provide you with high fiber, you must restrict these items. For 1-cup servings, these are the average carbs spent:

- Black beans: 41 grams of carbs (15 g fiber)
- Kidney beans: 40 grams of carbs (13 g fiber)
- Pinto beans: 45 grams of carbs (15 g fiber)
- Lentils: 40 grams of carbs (16 g fiber)
- Peas: 25 grams of carbs (9 g fiber)
- Chickpeas: 45 grams of carbs (12 g fiber)

Avoid pasta: Pasta is unbelievably high in carbohydrates. Just 1 cup of cooked pasta can reach 43 carbs (3 g fiber). Whole wheat improves the rate but is still 37 grams (6 g fiber). Have a dish of shirataki or spiralized zoodles (zucchini noodles).

Avoid bread & grains: Many cultures depend on bread from bagels to bread loaves, rolls, flatbreads, and tortillas. Take note that even 2 slices of bread can take you over your daily limit! It is difficult to believe, but these are the facts:

- Bagel – (1) 3-inch is 29 grams of carbs (1 g fiber)
- Whole – wheat bread – 1 slice is 17 grams of carbs (2 g fiber)
- White bread – 1 slice is 14 grams of carbs (1 g fiber)

- Flour tortilla – 10-inch: 36 grams of carbs (2 g fiber

Honey & sugars to avoid: Maltose, dextrose, honey, corn syrup, and maltodextrin should be avoided on the keto plan. These are how you could spend needless carbs:

- Honey: 17 g carbs
- Agave nectar: 16 g carbs
- White sugar: 12.6 g carbs
- Maple syrup: 13 g carbs

Artificial sweeteners: You should avoid Splenda, saccharin, and sucralose sweeteners.

Sugary foods: Leave the usual 'junk foods' alone including soda, many fruit juices, cake, ice cream, and candy. These are just a few examples of processed snacks to avoid while on a ketogenic diet. Some are surprising because they were deemed for years as a healthy snack. Do you recognize any of them?

- Protein Bars
- Cereal Bars
- Popcorn
- Rice cakes
- Flavored Nuts
- Potato Chips
- Pretzels
- Protein Bars
- Crackers

If you see carrageenan on the label, it is best to leave it on the shelf. It is an extract from red seaweed which is also known as Irish Moss. It has been used traditionally for hundreds of years. It is found in cottage cheese, non-dairy milk, pudding, jelly, and ice cream among others.

Don't feel too guilty if you crave all of those processed foods. It's normal. As a rule of thumb, look for labels with the least amount of ingredients. Usually, the ones that provide the most nutrition are listed in those 'short' lists.

Alcoholic Beverages & Your Ketogenic Status

Okay, so you are going to drink alcohol. Just remember, that alcohol is a controversial subject when it comes to a dieting plan. This isn't an endorsement for you to consume alcohol. However, the alcohol does produce ketones in the liver. It has been noted that people who drink alcohol are possibly more sensitive to the side effects while in ketosis, meaning, so if you drive, watch your limits closely.

Avoid cocktails, flavored liquor, and wine to remain in ketosis. You should also avoid mixers including soda, juices, or syrup. Note: Some professionals believe it is acceptable to drink these keto-friendly choices on special occasions:

- Bloody Mary for 5 grams
- Gin Rickey for 1.5 grams
- Manhattan for 2 grams
- Dry Martini Cocktail for 0 grams

Choose from these types of liquor to remain in ketosis:

- Vodka: Check the carb content since it is usually produced (grain-based) from rye, potatoes, and wheat.
- Tequila: The agave plant is the source for tequila. Mescal is a good option.
- Whiskey: Barley, corn, and rye are the grains used 0 - carbs or sugar.
- Rum: Choose the ones with zero carbs and no added sugar.
- Dry Sparkling Wine or Champagne: 1 serving is about 1 gram

- Dry White or Red Wine: 1 glass about 2 grams

You should also avoid beer since on average for a 12. oz serving for the following brands, you may be surprised:

- Busch Light, Lite, and Natural lite are the least at 3.2 grams of carbohydrates. Bud Ice is 4 grams with Coors Light rating 5 total grams.
- Ranking at 11 grams is Heineken, Budweiser, Becks, and others.
- Corona and Guinness rank at 14 grams.

The main point is that you do not compensate from those liquid carbs by eating less later. It's all up to you, just count the carbs. Also remember, the 'hangover' will also most likely be worse. So remember to drink plenty of water.

Chapter 3:

Adapt to a Ketogenic Lifestyle & Meal Prep

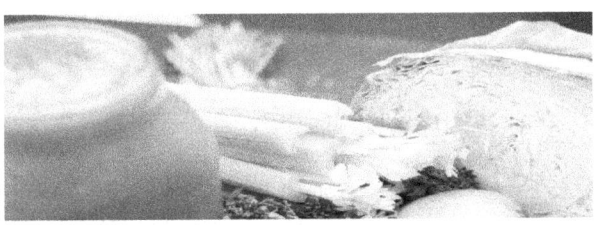

LIVING A KETOGENIC LIFESTYLE

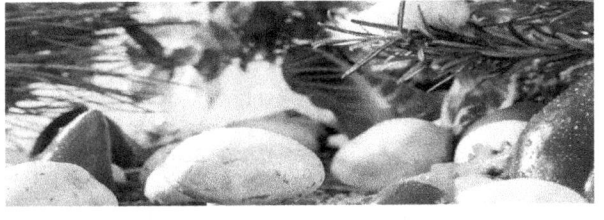

You will be able to adapt to your Keto lifestyle without sacrificing your freedom.

Understanding the Macronutrients or Macros

The first step is understanding the macronutrients and how they're calculated.

The macronutrients are building blocks of food consisting of protein, fat, and carbs. You will need to try one of the apps discussed later to discover what your 'keto numbers' are for daily consumption since each individual has a different amount allowed because of specific elements.

Maintain your weight with a balance of high fats and low carbs. To achieve weight loss, you will need to reduce your carbohydrate intake. The ketogenic techniques will provide you with the required foods to lose weight and not be hungry. Macros are found in varying amounts which are measured using grams. For example, fat equals approximately 9 calories per gram, protein at 4 calories, and the carbs at 4 calories for each gram.

Count the Calories or Micros: Which is Best?

The short of counting calories is that they don't tell the whole story. You can fill up on the 'right' calories and you may also lose muscle mass. For example, you count 100 calories of avocado which is a fat which is better than a 100-calorie cookie (carbs). That is why keto counts the macros (fat, protein, and carbs) not the calories.

Remember this formula: You will need to calculate your net carbs on some of the recipes you discover on the Internet — some list only the total carbs. If that happens, just take the total carbs listed (-) fiber (=) the total net carbs which is what you need to track for an accurate count so you can remain in ketosis.

How to Begin Prep

Meal prep might seem a bit challenging at first but just remember – you don't need to prep all of your meals at one time. You can begin with the meats one evening and veggies the next; it's all up to you! The segment using veggies in this book are prepared to use within a couple of days (unless otherwise shown).

Decide how to prep. Do you want to prepare all of the chicken, pork, or other meal selections one night and the veggies the next night? Or do you want to cook each meal individually but in bulk? No worries, either way since each of the recipes have instructions for individual prep tips as well.

Purchase or prepare the containers you want to use. These are some guidelines for those:

- Mason Jars – Pint or quart sized
- Ziploc – type freezer bags
- Rubbermaid Stackable – Glad Containers

  - ➢ Freezer Safe
  - ➢ Microwavable
  - ➢ BPA Free
  - ➢ Reusable
  - ➢ Stackable

Select a non-busy preparation day: Choose a time when you won't have any interruptions.

Make a current inventory of the pantry and other food storage areas: Purchase your food items in bulk to save money. Saving money while on the ketogenic diet is vital. Purchasing your items in bulk can make a severe impact. Shop around and explore your areas for stores such as Walmart, Costco, or Sam's Club. These stores generally have bargain prices. Check your area for local farms who raise their animals on pasture feeding or a local market for fresh produce. After you find a good deal, stock up and purchase pantry items such as seasonings and flour. You can freeze many things and save a bundle of cash.

Guidelines for Dairy - Meats & Veggies

Purchase whole - not chopped meats & veggies: You can save big by chopping or dicing your own meats and vegetables. You will pay for the person that is doing the cutting for your convenience.

Choose fresh meats and dairy when possible: Try to find meat and dairy that has an expiration date for as far in the future as possible. These choices will tend to remain fresh and last longer. This also applies to the "sell by" dates. The further in the future, either of these dates is, the surer you can be that the food is going to last the week.

Choose the menu plan: Gather your favorite recipes or try some new ones.

Choose a meal plan: To Follow

Consider these additional tips:

➤ Chop your veggies in advance.

➤ Prepare and freeze plenty of healthy fruits and yogurt into a delicious smoothie for the entire week. Enjoy one for breakfast or any time you have the craving.

➤ Purchase foods in bulk to be used for taco meats, breakfast burritos, fajita fillings, soups, egg muffins, and so much more.

➤ As you prep, include lean proteins for the weekends in a container for a quick grab 'n' go snack or luncheon for a weekend journey.

How to freeze & reheat your meats:

For meals that are scheduled to be eaten at least three days after cooking, freezing is a great option. Freezing food is safe and convenient, but it doesn't work for every type of meal. You can also freeze the ingredients for a slow cooker meal and then just dump out the container into the slow cooker and leave it there. This saves a lot of time and means you can pre-prep meals up to 1-2 months in advance.

The last food safety consideration you need to make with regards to meal prepping is how you reheat food. Most people opt to microwave their meals for warming, but you can use any other conventional heating source in your kitchen as well. The reason people love the microwave for heating their meal prep meals is that it's quick and convenient.

However, you have to be careful with microwaving because over-cooking can cause food to taste bad. To combat this, cook your food in one-minute intervals and check on it between each minute. You can also help your food cook more evenly and quickly but keeping your meat cut into small pieces when you cook it. You should never put food directly from the freezer into the microwave. Let your frozen food thaw first.

Food reheating and prep safety will become second nature over time. Meal prep can be overwhelming and require a lot of thought and patience, but it becomes a lot easier once you get used to it. Many of the mistakes are easy to avoid.

However, mistakes do happen, and as such, it's best to cook for short periods of time rather than longer ones, so you have less of a risk of making a mistake and needing to scrap everything you have prepared for that substantial period of time. While it is a lot and seems complicated, meal prepping is the best way to set yourself up for success with the keto diet.

Don't store hot food in the fridge: Keep your refrigerator at a proper temperature (should be below 40°F). If your refrigerator is warmer than this, it promotes the growth of bacteria. Any drastic temperature changes will cause condensation to form on the food items. You need to let your prepared food cool down in the open air before putting it in a container and closing the lid. The increased moisture levels can open the door to bacteria growth.

Label the containers: There are some other things you have to consider when freezing your meals. You should always label your container with the date that you put it in the freezer. You also need to double check that your bottles, jars, or bags are each sealed tightly. If your containers aren't air-tight, your food will become freezer burnt and need to be trashed.

Chapter 4

Meal Prep: The 21-Day Plan

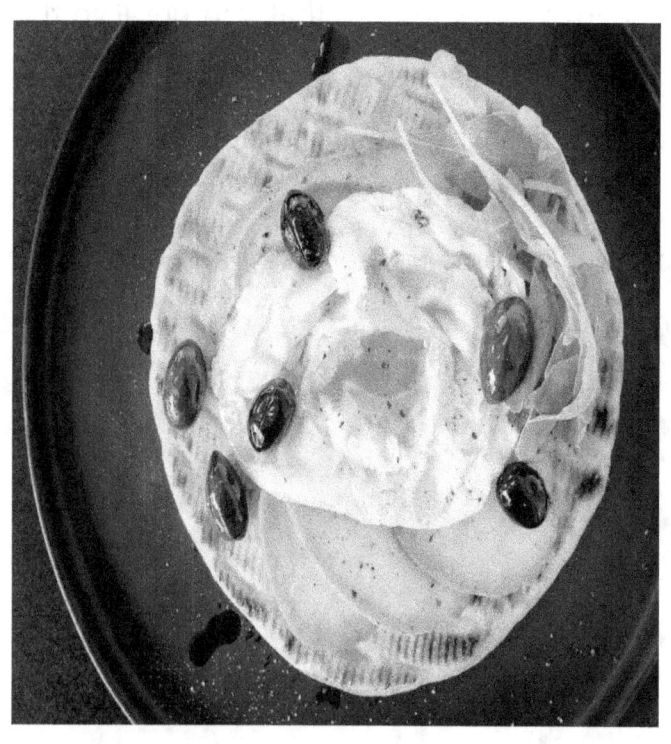

Each of these recipes has the net carbs per serving posted. You will see how flexible the plan is when you look at how easy it is to use just the recipes in this cookbook for 21 full days including 3 meals and snacks or desserts. The meals are planned so you still have flexibility in your eating patterns with extra carbs to use as desired. Even on the strictest diet plan, most of these recipes should be just what the doctor ordered. Calculate how many carbs you are allowed each day and add some healthy snacks or sides to these totals. It's all up to you, just track everything.

Week 1: Day 1

- **Breakfast:** Avocado & Eggs: 9 g Net Carbs
- **Lunch:** Chili Lime Cod: 3 g
- **Dinner:** Tasty Short Ribs: 2.5 g Net Carbs
- **Side Dish:** Caprese Salad: 5 g
- **Snacks:** Lemonade Fat Bombs: 7 g Net Carbs

Daily Total Net Carbs: 26.5

Week 1: Day 2

- **Breakfast:** Pancakes & Nuts: 9 g Net Carbs
- **Lunch:** Rainbow Salad: 1 g Net Carbs
- **Dinner:** Chicken & Gravy: 4 g Net Carbs
- **Side Dish:** Lemony Green Beans with Almonds: 6.5 g
- **Snacks:** Vanilla Cinnamon Protein Bites: 4 g Net Carbs

Daily Total Net Carbs: 24.5

Week 1: Day 3

- **Breakfast:** Bacon Cheese & Egg Cups: 1 g Net Carbs
- **Lunch:** BBQ Meat Lover's Pizza: 3.5 g Net Carbs
- **Dinner:** Pan-Fried Pork Chops: 4 g Net Carbs
- **Side Dish:** Lemony Green Beans with Almonds: 6.5 g
- **Snacks:** Spice Cakes: 3 g Net Carbs

Daily Total Net Carbs: 18

Week 1: Day 4

- **Breakfast:** Apple Banana Muffins: 8 g Net Carbs
- **Lunch:** Zoodle Chicken Soup: 4 g Net Carbs
- **Dinner:** Tasty Short Ribs: 2.5 g Net Carbs
- **Side Dish:** Baked Radishes & Brown Butter Sauce: 2 g
- **Snacks:** Brownie Muffins: 4.4 g Net Carbs

Daily Total Net Carbs: 20.9

Week 1: Day 5

Breakfast: Baked Greek Eggs: 5 g Net Carbs

Lunch: Italian Tomato Salad: 6 g Net Carbs

Dinner: Chicken and Asparagus Pan Dinner: 4 g Net Carbs

Snacks: Vanilla Cinnamon Protein Bites: 4 g Net Carbs

Daily Total Net Carbs: 19

Week 1: Day 6

- Breakfast: Blueberry Pancake Bites: 7.5 g Net Carbs
- Lunch: Zoodle Chicken Soup: 4 g Net Carbs
- Dinner: Authentic Butter Chicken: 6 g Net Carb
- Side Dish: Baked Radishes & Brown Butter Sauce: 2 g Net Carbs
- Snacks: Mocha Cheesecake Bars: 3 g Net Carbs

Daily Total Net Carbs: 22.5

Week 1: Day 7

- **Breakfast:** French Style Crepes: 5 g Net Carbs
- **Lunch:** Zoodle Chicken Soup: 4 g Net Carbs
- **Dinner:** Cumin Spiced Beef Wraps: 4 g Net Carbs
- **Snacks:** Cinnamon Apples – Instant Pot: 2 g Net Carbs

Daily Total Net Carbs: 15

Week 2: Day 1

- **Breakfast:** Spinach Quiche: 0 g Net Carbs
- **Lunch:** Beef & Pepperoni Pizza: 2 g Net Carbs
- **Dinner:** Asian-Inspired Pork Chops: 3 g Net Carbs
- **Side Dish:** Hibachi Mushrooms – Japanese Style: 3 g
- **Snacks:** Peanut Butter Protein Bars: 3 g Net Carbs

Daily Total Net Carbs: 11

Week 2: Day 2

- **Breakfast:** Cheddar-Jalapeno Waffles: 6 Net Carbs
- **Lunch:** Cauliflower & Citrus Salad: 1 g Net Carbs
- **Dinner:** Chicken Kiev: 4 g Net Carbs
- **Side Dish:** Hibachi Mushrooms – Japanese Style: 3 g
- **Snacks:** Peanut Butter Fudge: 0 g Net Carbs

Daily Total Net Carbs: 14

Week 2: Day 3

- **Breakfast:** Almost Mc Griddle Casserole: 3 g Net Carbs
- **Lunch:** Almond Pesto Salmon: 6 g
- **Dinner:** Sweet & Sour Meatballs: 5 g Net Carbs
- **Snacks:** Brownie Muffins: 4.4 g Net Carbs

Daily Total Net Carbs: 18.4

Week 2: Day 4

- **Breakfast:** French Style Crepes: 5 g Net Carbs
- **Lunch:** Beef & Pepperoni Pizza: 2 g Net Carbs
- **Dinner:** Chicken Parmesan: 3 g Net Carbs
- Side Dish: Cobb Salad: 3 g
- **Snacks:** Peanut Butter Protein Bars: 3 g Net Carbs

Daily Total Net Carbs: 16

Week 2: Day 5

- **Breakfast:** Pancakes & Nuts: 9 g Net Carbs
- **Lunch:** Caesar & Salmon Salad: 2 g Net Carbs
- **Dinner:** Balsamic Beef Pot Roast: 3 g Net Carbs
- **Side Dish:** Asparagus & Garlic: 2 g
- **Snacks:** Almond Butter Fat Bombs: 1.7 g Net Carbs

Daily Total Net Carbs: 17.7

Week 2: Day 6

- **Breakfast:** Tomato & Cheese Frittata: 6 g Net Carbs
- **Lunch:** Chicken Pot Pie Soup: 3.5 g Net Carbs
- **Dinner:** Parmesan Crusted Pork Chops: 3 g Net Carbs
- **Side Dish:** Cobb Salad: 3 g
- **Snacks:** Cheesecake Cupcakes: 2.1 g Net Carbs

Daily Total Net Carbs: 17.6

Week 2: Day 7

- **Breakfast:** Blueberry Pancake Bites: 7.5 g Net Carbs
- **Lunch:** Kale Salad: 3 g Net Carbs
- **Dinner:** Chicken & Bacon Patties: 1.5 g Net Carbs
- **Side Dish:** Asparagus & Garlic: 2 g
- **Snacks:** Blueberry Cream Cheese Fat Bombs: 1 g Net Carbs

Daily Total Net Carbs: 15

Week 3: Day 1

- **Breakfast:** Avocado & Eggs: 9 g Net Carbs
- **Lunch:** Beef & Pepperoni Pizza: 2 g Net Carbs
- **Dinner:** Pulled Pork: 2.2 g Net Carbs
- **Side Dish:** Caprese Salad: 5 g Net Carbs
- **Snacks:** Healthy Chia Bars: 1.5 g Net Carbs

Daily Total Net Carbs: 19.7

Week 3: Day 2

Breakfast: Baked Greek Eggs: 5 g Net Carbs

Lunch: Thai Pork Salad: 5 g Net Carbs

Dinner: Buffalo Chicken Burgers: 1 g Net Carbs

Side Dish: Buffalo Cauliflower Bites: 3 g

Snacks: Chocolate Fat Bombs: 1 g Net Carbs

Daily Total Net Carbs: 15

Week 3: Day 3

- **Breakfast:** Tomato & Cheese Frittata: 6 g
- **Lunch:** Creamy Salmon & Pasta: 3 g Net Carbs
- **Dinner:** Chicken Fried Pork Chops: 0.8 g Net Carbs
- **Side Dish:** Buffalo Cauliflower Bites: 3 g
- **Snacks:** Delicious No-Bake Coconut Cookies: 0 g Net Carbs

Daily Total Net Carbs: 12.8

Week 3: Day 4

- **Breakfast:** Almost Mc Griddle Casserole: 3 g Net Carbs
- **Lunch:** Pan-Fried Cod: 1 g Net Carbs
- **Dinner:** Chicken Parmesan: 3 g Net Carbs
- **Side Dish:** Cauliflower Mac & Cheese: 7 Net Carbs
- **Snacks:** Cheesecake Cupcakes: 2.1 g Net Carbs

Daily Total Net Carbs: 16.1

Week 3: Day 5

- **Breakfast:** Spinach Quiche: -0- g Net Carbs
- **Lunch:** Zoodle Chicken Soup: 4 g Net Carbs
- **Dinner:** Tasty Short Ribs: 2.5 Net Carbs
- **Side Dish:** Cauliflower Mac & Cheese: 7 Net Carbs
- **Snacks:** Peanut Butter Protein Bars: 3 g Net Carbs

Daily Total Net Carbs: 16.5

Week 3: Day 6

- **Breakfast:** Baked Greek Eggs: 5 g Net Carbs
- **Lunch:** BLT Salad: 7 g Net Carbs
- **Dinner:** Pulled Pork: 2.2 g Net Carbs
- **Side Dish:** Buffalo Cauliflower Bites: 3 g
- **Snacks:** Peanut Butter Fudge: 0 g Net Carbs

Daily Total Net Carbs: 17.2

Week 3: Day 7

- Breakfast: Bacon Cheese & Egg Cups: 1 g Net Carbs
- Lunch: Creamy Salmon & Pasta: 3 g Net Carbs
- Dinner: Chicken and Asparagus Pan Dinner: 4 g Net Carbs
- Snacks: Coffee Fat Bombs: -0- g Net Carbs

Daily Total Net Carbs: 8

Final Note: You can add additional snacks if you have not met your daily quotas.

Chapter 5

<u>Delicious Breakfast</u>

<u>Dishes</u>

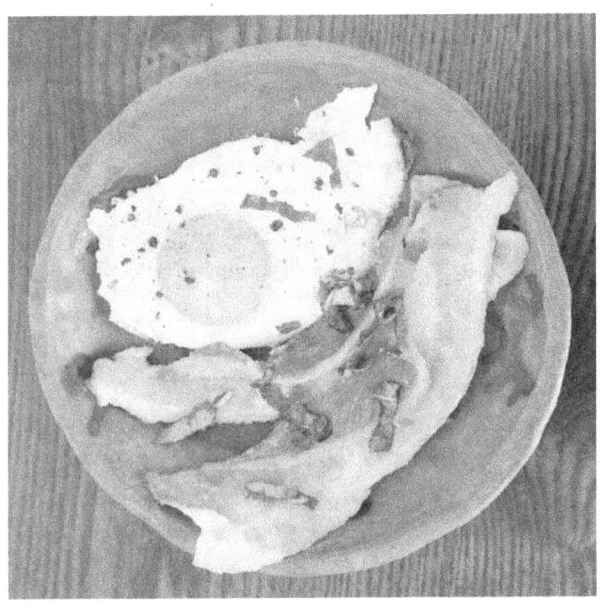

From eggs to sweet goodies, you are sure to find a perfect breakfast dish here!

Eggs Delight

Almost Mc Griddle Casserole

Serving Yields: 8

Macros: 3 g Net Carbs | 448 Calories | 26 g Protein | 36 g Total Fats

Fixings Needed:

- Breakfast sausage - 1 lb.
- Flaxseed meal - .25 cup
- Almond flour - 1 cup
- Large eggs - 10
- Maple syrup - 6 tbsp.
- Cheese - 4 oz.
- Butter - 4 tbsp.
- Onion - .5 tsp.
- Garlic powder - .5 tsp.
- Sage - .25 tsp.
- Also Needed: 9 x 9-inch casserole dish

How to Prepare:

1. Heat up the oven temperature to 350°F.

2. Use the medium heat setting on the stovetop to prepare the sausage in a skillet. Add all of the dry ingredients (the cheese also) and stir in the wet ones. Add 4 tablespoons of the syrup. Stir and blend well.

3. After the sausage is browned, combine all of the fixings along with the grease.

4. Prepare the casserole dish with a sheet of parchment paper. Empty the mix into the casserole dish and drizzle the rest of the syrup on the top.

5. Bake for 45-55 minutes.

6. Transfer to the countertop and let it become room temperature. The casserole should be easy to remove by using the edge of the parchment paper.

Meal Prep Tips:

1. After the casserole has cooled, just slice it into 8 portions.
2. You can enjoy for a couple of days.
3. You can also freeze the rest for later.

Avocado & Eggs

Serving Yields: 2

Macros: 9 g Net Carbs | 275 Calories | 8 g Protein | 23 g Total Fats

Fixings Needed:

- Eggs - 2
- Avocado - 1 ripened
- Optional: Hot sauce
- Salt & Freshly cracked black pepper - to your liking

How to Prepare:

1. Warm up the oven until it reaches 425°F.
2. Slice the avocado in half and discard the pit. Use a metal scoop to remove about 1-2 tablespoons of the fleshy insides.

Arrange the halves in a small baking pan. Crack an egg into both halves and season with some pepper and salt.

3. Bake 15-20 minutes.

Meal Prep Tips:

1. Let the fixings cool and store for a day or so in the refrigerator to enjoy the next morning or for a snack.
2. If you want to spice it up a little, sprinkle in a portion of keto-friendly hot sauce on the second day.

Bacon Cheese & Egg Cups

Serving Yields: 6

Macros: 1 g Net Carbs | 101 Calories | 8 g Protein | 7 g Total Fats

Fixings Needed:

- Large eggs - 6
- Bacon - 6 strips
- Cheese - .25 cup
- Fresh spinach - 1 handful
- Pepper & Salt - to taste

How to Prepare:

1. Warm up the oven to 400°F.
2. Prepare the bacon using medium heat on the stovetop. Place on towels to drain.
3. Grease 6 muffin tins with a spritz of oil.

4. Line each tin with a slice of bacon, pressing tightly to make a secure well for the eggs.
5. Drain and dry the spinach with a paper towel. Whisk the eggs and combine with the spinach.
6. Add the mixture to the prepared tins and sprinkle with cheese. Sprinkle with salt and pepper until it's like you like it.
7. Bake for 15 minutes. Remove when done and cool.

Meal Prep Tips:

1. Prepare the cups and store in airtight containers.
2. Reheat when ready to eat. It keeps in the fridge for 3-4 days.

Baked Greek Eggs

Servings: 6

Macros: 175 Calories | 5 g Net Carbs | 11 g Total Fats | 15 g Protein

Fixings Needed:

- Sun-dried tomatoes - .25 cup
- Feta cheese - .5 cup
- Oregano - .5 tsp.
- Chopped kale - 1 cup
- Eggs - 12

How to Prepare:

- Warm up the oven to reach 350ºF.
- Cover a baking tin with foil and a spritz of nonstick cooking spray.
- Whisk the eggs and combine with the rest of the fixings. Stir into the prepared pan. Bake for 25 minutes.

- Transfer to the countertop to completely cool. Slice.

Meal Prep Tips:

1. Store in the refrigerator for 4-5 days in an airtight container.
2. You can also place them into individual portions.

Spinach Quiche

Serving Yields: 6

Macros: -0- g Net Carbs | 299 Calories | 19.4 g Protein | 23 g Total Fats

Fixings Needed:

- Chopped onion - 1
- Olive oil - 1 tbsp.
- Frozen & thawed spinach - 1 pkg. 10 oz.
- Shredded Muenster cheese - 3 cups
- Organic eggs - whisked - 5
- To Taste: Black pepper and salt
- Also Needed: 9-inch pie plate

How to Prepare:

1. Warm up the oven to reach 350°F. Lightly grease the dish.

2. Use the medium heat setting to warm a skillet with the oil. Toss in the onion and sauté for 4-5 minutes. Raise the heat setting to medium-high.

3. Add the spinach and sauté for two to three minutes until the liquid is absorbed. Cool slightly

4. Combine the rest of the fixings in a large bowl and mix with the cooled spinach. Dump into the prepared dish and bake for 30 minutes.

5. Take the quiche out of the oven and cool for at least ten minutes.

6. Slice into six wedges.

Meal Prep Tips:

1. Add the cooled pieces into plastic baggies.
2. It will store in the fridge for two to four days.
3. To warm up, just prepare in the microwave for one minute on the high setting before serving.

Tomato & Cheese Frittata

Serving Yields: 2

Macros: 6 g Net Carbs | 435 Calories | 27 g Protein | 33 g Total Fats

Fixings Needed:

- Eggs - 6
- Soft cheese - 3.5 oz. - .66 cup
- White onion - .5 of 1 medium
- Halved cherry tomatoes - .66 cup
- Chopped herbs - ex. Chives or basil - 2 tbsp.
- Ghee or butter - 1 tbsp.

How to Prepare:

1. Set the oven broiler temperature to 400°F.
2. Arrange the onions on a greased - hot iron skillet. Cook with either the ghee or butter until lightly browned.
3. In another dish, crack the eggs and flavor with the salt, pepper, or add some herbs of your choice. Whisk and add to the pan of onions, cooking until the edges begin to get crispy.
4. Top with the cheese (such as feta) and a few diced tomatoes. Put the pan in the broiler for five to seven minutes or until done.
5. Enjoy piping hot or let cool down.
6. Note: You can purge all of the leftover veggies into the recipe (if you wish).

Meal Prep Tips:

1. Divide into two equal portions. Place in separate containers until you're ready to enjoy a healthy breakfast.
2. Enjoy this readily prepared frittata that you can serve either hot or cold.
3. The deliciously prepared frittata will store in the fridge for up to five days. So, prep enough for several days.

Other Delicious Choices

Apple Banana Muffins

Serving Yields: 12

Macros: 8 g Net Carbs | 134 Calories | 11 g Protein | 4 g Total Fats

Fixings Needed:

- Baking powder - 1 tsp.
- Salt - .25 tsp.
- Baking soda - .5 tsp.
- Egg - 1
- Olive oil - 3 tbsp.
- Vanilla extract - 1 tsp.
- Unsweetened applesauce - .5 cup
- Ripe bananas - 1.5 cups
- Whole wheat flour - 1.33 cups

How to Prepare:

1. Heat up the oven to 375ºF. Heavily grease a muffin tin.
2. Whisk the egg and add the mashed bananas. Stir in everything but the flour.
3. Next, fold in the flour, being careful not to overmix. Pour into the muffin tin and bake for approximately 20-25 minutes.

Meal Prep Tips:

1. When the muffins are done, transfer them to the countertop and cool in the pan for about 5 minutes. At that time, arrange them on a cooling rack to thoroughly cool before proceeding.
2. Place the muffins in a storage container or freezer baggie.
3. Store in the fridge for about 5 days or freeze for later.

Blueberry Pancake Bites

Serving Yields: 24 bites

Macros: 7.5 g Net Carbs | 188 Calories | 6 g Protein | 13 g Total Fats

Fixings Needed:

- Baking powder - 1 tsp
- Water - .33 - .5 cup
- Melted ghee - .25 cup
- Coconut flour - .5 cup
- Cinnamon - .5 tsp.
- Salt - .5 tsp.
- Eggs - 4
- Vanilla extract - .5 tsp.
- Frozen blueberries - .5 cup
- Also Needed: Muffin tray

How to Prepare:

1. Warm up the oven to reach 325°F. Use a spritz of coconut oil spray to grease 24 muffin cups.

2. Combine the eggs, sweetener, and vanilla; mixing until smooth. Fold in the flour, melted ghee, salt, baking powder, and cinnamon. Stir in .33 cup of water to finish the batter.

3. The mixture should be thick. Next, divide the batter into the prepared cups with several berries in each one.

4. Bake until set (20-25 min.). Cool.

Meal Prep Tips:

1. Store in an airtight container, preferably cool also.

2. It will be good for 8-10 days.

3. Freeze for 60-80 days.

Cheddar-Jalapeno Waffles

Serving Yields: 1

Macros: 6 g Net Carbs | 338 Calories | 16 g Protein | 28 g Total Fats

Fixings Needed:

- Large eggs - 3
- Jalapeno - 1 small
- Cream cheese - 3 oz.
- Coconut flour - 1 tbsp.
- Cheddar cheese - 1 oz.
- Baking powder - 1 tsp.
- Psyllium husk powder - 1 tsp.

How to Prepare:

1. Mix all of the ingredients using an immersion blender except for the jalapeno and cheese.

2. After you have a smooth texture, add the cheese and jalapeno. Blend and pour the batter into the waffle iron.
3. Cook for 5-6 minutes. Set aside when done.

Meal Prep Tips:

1. Let the waffles cool off for prep.
2. Put them into a plastic freezer bag. Store them in the freezer until you have the desire for a delicious waffle.
3. To reheat, preheat the oven temperature to 400ºF. When it's hot, place the waffles on a baking tin. Warm them up for 5 minutes. Serve and enjoy!
4. Tip: It isn't recommended to warm them in a regular toaster.

Note: These delicious waffles are complemented by psyllium husk which is a native of Pakistan, Bangladesh, and India. Its fiber content is right for your gut as a bulk-forming laxative which is useful in the keto diet since constipation can be one of the side effects.

French Style Crepes

Serving Yields: 2

Macros: 5 g Net Carbs | 319 Calories | 8 g Protein | 27.4 g Total Fats

Fixings Needed:

- Organic eggs - 2
- Melted coconut oil - divided – 2 tbsp.
- Sea salt - .125 tsp.
- Splenda - 1 tsp.
- Coconut flour - 2 tbsp.
- Heavy cream - .33 cup

How to Prepare:

1. Whisk the eggs, 1 tablespoon of oil, salt, and Splenda.

2. Slowly add the flour, whisking until well mixed. Stir in the cream.

3. Use the rest of the oil to grease a pan. Empty in 1/4 of the mixture and tilt the skillet to make a thin layer. Cook for two minutes, flip, and cook one more minute.

4. Proceed with the rest of the egg mixture to make the four crepes. Cool thoroughly.

Meal Prep Tips:

1. Wrap each one in plastic. Store in the fridge for up to two days.

2. Simply reheat in the microwave for 30 seconds when ready to use.

Pancakes & Nuts

Serving Yields: 2

Macros: 9 g Net Carbs | 625 Calories | 27 g Protein | 52 g Total Fats

Fixings Needed:

- Almond flour - 10 tbsp.
- Ground cinnamon - 1 tsp.
- Baking soda - .5 tsp.
- Large eggs - 3
- Almond milk - .25 cup
- Chopped nuts - ex. Hazelnuts – .25 cup
- Unsweetened almond/preference nut butter - .25 cup

How to Prepare:

1. Whisk all of the fixings in a container. Let the batter sit for 5-10 minutes so the flour will thicken.
2. Warm up a greased skillet (low-medium).
3. Measure out .25 cup portions of the batter in the frying pan. Cook for 2-3 minutes per side.

Meal Prep Tips:

1. Let the pancakes cool.
2. Pour the nuts into a baggie or plastic container. You can add the nuts in the containers together or separately.
3. You can store the pancakes for 5-7 days in the refrigerator.
4. Time to Eat: Warm up the pancakes and serve with the prepared almond butter drizzle.

Keto-Friendly Breakfast Beverages

These two options are a great incentive to get going with your meal prep, so just enjoy!

Bulletproof Coffee

Serving Yields: 1

Macros: 0 g Net Carbs | 320 Calories | 1 g Protein | 51 g Total Fats

Fixings Needed:

- MCT oil powder - 2 tbsp.
- Ghee/butter - 2 tbsp.
- Hot coffee - 1.5 cups

How to Prepare:

1. Empty the hot coffee into your blender.
2. Pour in the powder and butter. Blend until frothy.
3. Enjoy using a large mug.

Avocado Mint Green Smoothie

Serving Yields: 1

Macros: 5 g Net Carbs | 223 Calories | 1 g Protein |23 g Total Fats

Fixings Needed:

- Almond milk - .5 cup
- Full-fat coconut milk - .75 cup
- Avocado - .5 of 1 – approx. 3-4 oz.
- Cilantro - 3 sprigs
- Large mint leaves - 5-6
- Vanilla extract - .25 tsp.
- Lime juice - 1 squeeze
- Sweetener of your choice - to your liking
- Crushed ice - 1.5 cup

How to Prepare:

1. Measure each of the ingredients and add to your blender.
2. Combine on the low-speed setting until pureed.

Meal Prep Tips:

1. At this point, you can store in the fridge.
2. When you are ready to have the smoothie, just toss in the ice and mix.
3. Serve in a cold glass.

Blueberry Essence

Serving Yields: 1

Macros: 3 g Net Carbs | 343 Calories | 31 g Protein | 21 g Total Fats

Fixings Needed:

- Blueberries - .25 cup
- Coconut milk - 1 cup
- Whey protein powder (optional) - 1 scoop
- Vanilla Essence - 1 tsp.
- MCT Oil - 1 tsp.

How to Prepare:

1. For a quick burst of energy, add all of the fixings into a blender.
2. Puree until it reaches the desired consistency.

Meal Prep Tips:

1. Store in the fridge until ready to enjoy.
2. Add several chunks of ice if you like.

Blueberry Yogurt Smoothie

Serving Yields: 2

Macros: 2 g Net Carbs | 70 Calories | 2 g Protein | 5 g Total Fats

Fixings Needed:

- Blueberries - 10
- Yogurt - .5 cup
- Vanilla extract - .5 tsp.
- Coconut milk - 1 cup
- Stevia - to your liking

How to Prepare:

1. Add all of the fixings into the blender, mixing well.
2. When creamy, pour into 2 chilled mugs and enjoy.

Cinnamon Smoothie

Serving Yields: 1

Macros: 5 g Net Carbs | 467 Calories | 24 g Protein | 40.3 g Total Fats

Fixings Needed:

- Cinnamon - .5 tsp.
- Coconut milk - .5 cup
- Water - .5 cup
- Extra-virgin coconut oil/MCT oil - 1 tbsp.
- Ground chia seeds - 1 tbsp.
- Plain/vanilla whey protein - .25 cup
- Stevia drops - optional

How to Prepare:

1. Pour the milk, cinnamon, protein powder, and chia seeds in a blender.
2. Empty the coconut oil, ice, and water. Add a few drops of stevia to your liking.

Chapter 6:

Tempting Lunchtime Choices

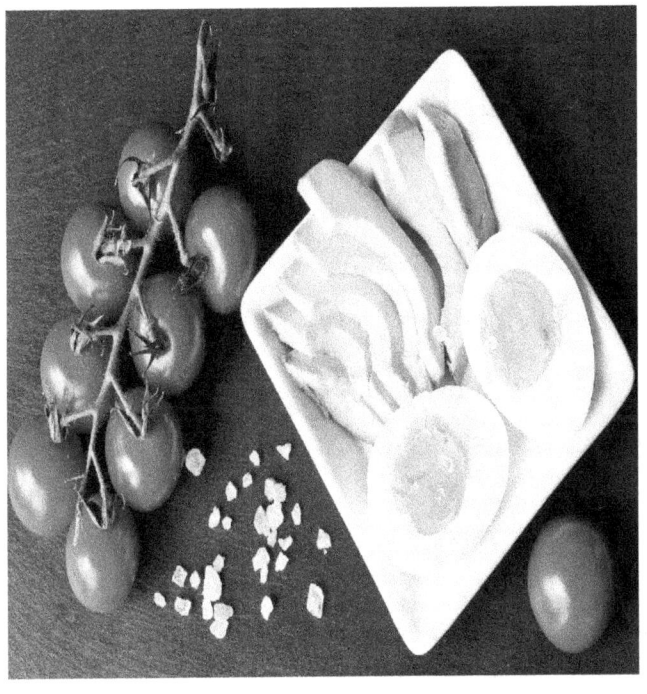

You have a wide variety to choose from, ranging from salads to soup and more.

Salad Choices

BLT Salad in a Jar

Serving Yields: 8

Macros: 7 g Net Carbs | 205 Calories | 17 g Protein |18 g Total Fats

Fixings Needed:

- Romaine Lettuce – 2 cups
- Iceberg Lettuce – 2 cups
- Chopped scallions – 2
- Diced tomatoes – 2
- Bacon slices – 4 crumbled

How to Prepare:

1. Combine all of the dressing ingredients.
2. Slowly pour into the jars.
3. Layer the veggies, croutons, and garnish of bacon.

Meal Prep Tips:

1. Tightly close each of the jars.
2. Store in the fridge for up to three days.

Caesar & Salmon Salad

Serving Yields: 2

Macros: 2 g Net Carbs | 466 Calories | 40 g Protein |32 g Total Fats

Fixings Needed:

- Salmon fillets – 2 – 6 oz. ea.
- Bacon – 4 slices
- Ghee – as needed – 1 tbsp.
- Freshly cracked black pepper – 1 pinch
- Pink salt – 1 pinch
- Sliced avocado – .5 of 1
- Romaine hearts – 2 cups chopped
- Caesar dressing – 2 tbsp.

How to Prepare:

1. Cook the bacon until crispy for 8 minutes using the med-high heat setting on the stovetop. Drain on a platter using paper towels.
2. Remove the excess water from the fillets. Give them a shake of pepper and salt.
3. Use the same pan to prepare the salmon. Add butter if needed.
4. Cook for five minutes per side. This will be medium-rare.
5. Break the bacon into bits.

Meal Prep Tips:

1. Prepare two salad dishes or closed container for the meal prep with equal parts of romaine, avocado, and the bacon.

2. Place the bacon into separate containers to keep them crunchy.
3. When ready to serve, enjoy with a drizzle of the dressing.

Cauliflower & Citrus Salad

Serving Yields: 4

Macros: 1 Net Carbs | 177 Calories | 2 g Protein | 7 g Total Fats

Fixings Needed for the Salad:

- Small cauliflower – 1 - divided
- Small Romanesco cauliflower – 1 - divided
- Broccoli – 1 lb.
- Seedless oranges – 2

Fixings Needed for the Vinaigrette:

- Finely chopped anchovies – 4
- Orange – juice & zest – 1
- Salted – unrinsed capers – 1 tbsp.
- Finely chopped hot pepper – 1
- Pepper & Salt – to your liking

- Extra-virgin olive oil – 4 tbsp.

How to Prepare:

1. Cut the cauliflower into florets. Remove the peel and thinly slice the oranges. Finely chop the anchovies, capers, and hot peppers for the vinaigrette.
2. Prepare the vinaigrette fixings in a jar with a lid. Shake well and set aside.
3. Set up the Instant Pot with one cup of water and the steamer basket. Add the cauliflower to the basket and secure the lid. Set the timer for 6 minutes using low pressure. Quick-release the steam pressure when you hear the buzzer.
4. Transfer the florets to a serving dish with the prepared oranges. Toss.
5. Drizzle with the vinaigrette and enjoy.

Meal Prep Tips:

1. Prepare the salad and dressing.
2. Store in the fridge individually or in a large air-tight container.

Italian Tomato Salad

Serving Yields: 2

Macros: 6 g Net Carbs | 274 Calories | 14.1 g Protein | 22 g Total Fats

Fixings Needed:

- Minced garlic clove – 1
- Freshly chopped basil – .25 cup
- Olive oil – 2 tbsp.
- Balsamic vinegar – 1 tbsp.
- Pepper and salt – to taste
- Sliced ripe tomatoes – 2 Medium
- Fresh arugula – 3 cups
- Cubed mozzarella cheese – 3 oz.

How to Prepare:

1. Combine the oil, basil, garlic pepper, salt, and vinegar in a blender. Mix until smooth.
2. Toss the rest of the fixings in a salad container.

Meal Prep Tips:

Combine the salad and add the dressing mixture or add it to individual containers for an on-to-go method.

You can store this way for up to one day.

Kale Salad

Serving Yields: 4

Macros: 3 g Net Carbs | 80 Calories| 4 g Protein |6 g Total Fats

Fixings Needed:

- Kale – 1 bunch
- Lemon juice – 1 tbsp.
- Extra-virgin olive oil – 1 tbsp.
- Salt – .5 tsp.
- Parmesan cheese – .33 cup

How to Prepare:

1. Cut away the ribs from the kale and slice into ¼-inch strips. Store in a plastic bag or storage container until ready to eat.

Meal Prep Tips:

2. When you're ready to eat, just combine with the salt and oil, toss about 3 minutes until softened.
3. Combine the cheese, juice, and kale. Serve.

Rainbow Salad

Serving Yields: 8

Macros: 1 g Net Carbs |109 Calories | 15 g Protein | 9 g Total Fats

Fixings Needed for the Dressing:

- White balsamic vinegar – .5 cup
- Olive oil – 2 tbsp.
- Minced garlic cloves – 2
- Chopped parsley – .25 cup
- Salt & Pepper – 1 pinch

Fixings Needed for the Salad:

- Chopped red cabbage – 2 cups
- Assorted salad greens – 8 cups
- Chopped cucumber – 1 cup
- Sliced carrots – 1 cup

- Raw sunflower seeds – .5 cup
- Diced red bell pepper – 1
- Chopped yellow pepper – 1

How to Prepare:

1. Whisk all of the dressing fixings together. Pour into a serving container.
2. Drain the chickpeas and prep the veggies. Prepare the salads.

Meal Prep Tips:

1. You can refrigerate the salad for up to five days.
2. Pour the dressing into a closed jar and place in the fridge until it is dinner or lunch time.

3. Another Option: You can also add the dressing in the bottom of a mason jar with the salad fixings on top.

Time to Eat: Put the salad in individual dishes and pour on the dressing. If you used a jar, just shake and enjoy!

Thai Pork Salad

Serving Yields: 2

Macros: 5 g Net Carbs | 461 Calories | 29 g Protein | 33 g Total Fats

Fixings Needed for the Sauce:

- Juice & zest of 1 lime
- Chopped cilantro – 2 tbsp.
- Tomato paste – 2 tbsp.
- Soy sauce – 2 tbsp (+) 2 tsp.
- Red curry paste – 1 tsp.
- Five Spice – 1 tsp.
- Fish sauce – 1 tsp.
- Red pepper flakes – .25 tsp.
- Rice wine vinegar – 1 tbsp. (+) 1 tsp.
- Mango extract – .5 tsp.
- Liquid stevia – 10 drops

Fixings Needed for the Salad:

- Romaine lettuce – 2 cups
- Pulled pork – 10 oz.
- Medium chopped red bell pepper – .25 of 1
- Chopped cilantro – .25 cup

How to Prepare:

1. Zest half of the lime and chop the cilantro.
2. Mix all of the sauce fixings.
3. Blend the barbecue sauce components and set aside.
4. Pull the pork apart and make the salad. Pour a glaze over the pork with a bit of the sauce.

Meal Prep Tips:

1. Prepare the salad and sauce fixings.
2. Prepare the pork and shred.
3. Store in individual containers or in the fridge to use within a day or so.

Tuna Salad

Serving Yields: 2

Macros: 6 g Net Carbs | 465 Calories | 68.5 g Protein |18 g Total Fats

Fixings Needed:

- Fresh lemon juice – .5 of 1
- Olive oil – 1 tbsp.
- Large chopped boiled eggs – 2
- Tuna packed in oil – 2 cans – 15 oz.
- Sliced cucumber – .5 of 1
- Medium red onions – thinly sliced - 2
- Cilantro – .5 of 1
- Salt – 1 tsp.
- Dijon mustard – 2 tsp.
- Mayonnaise – 2 tbsp.

Meal Prep Tips:

1. Whisk the oil, lemon juice, mayo, and mustard in a container.
2. Drain the tuna and combine with the remainder the ingredients in another bowl.
3. Place each container in the fridge.
4. Ready to Eat: Add the dressing to the salad and toss to serve.

Soups

Chicken Pot Pie Soup

Serving Yields: 6

Macros: 3.5 g Net Carbs | 432 Calories | 20.5 g Protein |35 g Total Fats

Fixings Needed:

- Butter – 2 tbsp.
- Skinless – boneless chicken breasts – 1-1.5 lb.
- Small diced onion – .25 of 1
- Mixed veggies – .5 cup
- Chicken broth – 3 cups
- Black pepper – .25 tsp.
- Pink salt – .25 tsp.
- Minced cloves of garlic – 2
- Heavy whipping cream – 1.75 cups

- Cream cheese – 1 oz.
- Rosemary – .25 tsp
- Poultry seasoning – 1 tsp.
- Thyme – 1 pinch
- Xanthan gum – .5 tsp.

How to Prepare:

1. Melt the butter in the Instant Pot using the saute mode. Toss in the mixed veggies and onion. Cook a few minutes until translucent. Add them to a bowl and set to the side.
2. Deglaze the Instant Pot with 1/2 c. of the broth. Toss in the chicken along with the spices.
3. Close the top and select the poultry setting (15 min.). Natural release for six minutes and do a quick release of the rest of the pressure.

4. Shred the chicken and add the rest of the broth, chicken, cream cheese, veggies, and whipping cream into the pot.
5. Switch to the warm cycle and add the xanthan gum. Stir and saute about 10 minutes.

Meal Prep Tips:

1. Be sure to cool down the fixings completely.
2. Either store them in a covered glass dish or in individual dishes.
3. They will remain delicious for at least 2-3 days.

Zoodle Chicken Soup

Serving Yields: 2

Macros: 4 g Net Carbs | 310 Calories | 34 g Protein | 16 g Total Fats

Fixings Needed:

- Chicken broth – 3 cups
- Chicken breast – 1
- Avocado oil – 2 tbsp.
- Green onion – 1
- Celery stalk – 1
- Cilantro – .25 cup
- Salt – to taste
- Peeled zucchini – 1

How to Prepare:

1. Chop or dice the breast of the chicken. Pour the oil into a saucepan and cook the chicken until done. Pour in the broth and simmer. Chop the celery and green onions and toss into the pan. Simmer for 3-4 more minutes.

2. Chop the cilantro and prepare the zucchini noodles. Use a spiralizer or potato peeler to make the 'noodles.' Add to the pot.

3. Simmer for a few more minutes and season to your liking.

Meal Prep Tips:

1. Store in a glass container in the fridge. It will remain tasty for 2-3 days.

Pizza for Lunch

BBQ Meat-Lover's Pizza

Serving Yields: 2

Macros: 3.5 g Net Carbs | 18 g Protein | 27 g Total Fats

Fixings Needed:

- Mozzarella - 8 oz. – 2 cups
- Psyllium husk powder – 1 tbsp.
- Almond flour – .75 cup
- Cream cheese – 1.5 oz. - 3 tbsp.
- Large egg – 1
- Black pepper – .5 tsp
- Salt – .5 tsp.
- Italian seasoning – 1 tbsp.

Fixings Needed for the Topping:

- Mozzarella cheese – 4 oz. 1 cup
- BBQ sauce – to your liking
- Sliced Kabana/hard salami
- Bacon slices
- Sprinkled oregano – optional

How to Prepare:

2. Set the temperature of the oven to 400°F.
3. Melt the cheese in the microwave – about 45 seconds. Toss in the cream cheese and egg, mixing well.
4. Blend in the psyllium husk, flour, salt, pepper, and Italian seasoning. Make the dough as circular as possible. Bake for ten minutes. Flip it onto a piece of parchment paper.

5. Cover the crust with the toppings. Sprinkle with more cheese.
6. Bake until the cheese is golden.

Meal Prep Tips:

1. According to your taste, you can cool the pizza thoroughly and slice.
2. Place in a freezer bag either as a whole or individually (if it makes it that far).

Beef & Pepperoni Pizza

Serving Yields: 4

Macros: 2 g Net Carbs | 610 Calories | 44 g Protein | 45 g Total Fats

Fixings Needed:

- Large eggs – 2
- Ground beef – 20 oz.
- Pepperoni slices – 28
- Pizza sauce – .5 cup
- Shredded cheddar cheese – .5 cup
- Mozzarella cheese – 4 oz.
- Also Needed: 1 Cast iron skillet

How to Prepare:

1. Combine the eggs, beef, and seasonings and place in the skillet to form the crust. Bake until the meat is done or about 15 minutes.
2. Take it out of the oven and add the sauce, cheese, and toppings. Place the pizza back in the oven a few more minutes until the cheese has melted.

Meal Prep Tips:

1. After it's cooled completely, slice the pizza into four equal portions for freezing.
2. You can also leave it whole and freeze. Add to a freezer bag until it's time to serve and enjoy.

Pita Pizza

Serving Yields: 2

Macros: 4 g Net Carbs | 250 Calories | 13 g Protein | 19 g Total Fats

Fixings Needed:

- Marinara sauce – .5 cup
- Low-carb pita – 1
- Cheddar cheese – 2 oz.
- Pepperoni – 14 slices
- Roasted red peppers – 1 oz.

How to Prepare:

1. Set the oven to 450ºF.
2. Slice the pita in half and put on a foil-lined baking tray. Rub with a bit of oil and toast for one to two minutes.

3. Pour the sauce over the bread, sprinkle with the cheese, and other toppings. Bake for another five minutes or until the cheese melts.

Meal Pep Tips:

1. Remove from the oven and let it cool thoroughly.
2. Store in the fridge for a couple of days.
3. Freeze to enjoy later using a freezer bag.

Seafood for Lunch

Cod Choices

Chili Lime Cod

Serving Yields: 2

Macros: 3 g Net Carbs | 215 Calories | 37 g Protein | 5 g Total Fats

Fixings Needed:

- Wild-caught cod – 10-12 oz.
- Coconut flour – .33 cup
- Egg – 1
- Lime – 1
- Cayenne pepper – .5 tsp.
- Garlic powder – 1 tsp.
- Salt – 1 tsp.
- Crushed red pepper – 1 tsp.

How to Prepare:

1. Heat the oven temperature to reach 400°F.
2. In separate dishes, whip the egg and remove any lumps from the flour.
3. Let the fillet soak in the egg dish for one minute on each side. Add it to the flour dish and then add it to a baking sheet.
4. Sprinkle the spices and drizzle the lime juice over the cod.
5. Bake 10 to 12 minutes or when it easily flakes apart.

Meal Pep Tips:

1. Cool completely once it is like you like it.
2. Wrap well in foil and store in the fridge for a day.
3. Freeze and enjoy later.
4. Once it is time to eat, just drizzle with some Sriracha if you wish, and enjoy.

Pan Fried Cod

Serving Yields: 4

Macros: 1 g Net Carbs | 160 Calories |21 g Protein |7 g Total Fats

Fixings Needed:

- Ghee – 3 tbsp.
- Cod fillets – 4
- Minced garlic cloves – 6
- Garlic powder – shake
- Salt – 1 pinch

How to Prepare:

1. Melt the ghee and add half of the garlic into a skillet.
2. Arrange the fillets in the pan using med-high heat. Sprinkle with the garlic pepper and the salt.
3. Once it turns white halfway up its side, turn it over and add the remainder of the minced garlic. Continue cooking until it flakes easily.

Meal Prep Tips:

1. Store a day or so or wrap up in foil and add to a plastic freezer bag for a longer time.
2. When ready to eat, serve with some ghee/garlic from the pan.

Salmon

Almond Pesto Salmon

Serving Yields: 2

Macros: 6 g Net Carbs | 610 Calories | 38 g Protein | 47 g Total Fats

Fixings Needed:

- Garlic clove - 1
- Almonds - .25 cup
- Olive oil - 1 tbsp.
- Lemon - .5 of 1
- Parsley - .5 tsp.
- Pink Himalayan salt - .5 tsp.
- Atlantic salmon fillets - 2 - 6 oz.
- Shallot - .5 of 1
- Lettuce - 2 handfuls
- Butter - 2 tbsp.

How to Prepare:

1. Make the Pesto: Pulse the almonds, garlic, and olive oil in the food processor to form a paste. Add the parsley, salt, and juice of the lemon. Set to the side.

2. Dry the salmon fillets and season them with a sprinkle of salt and pepper.

3. Cook the salmon four to six minutes (skin side down) in a lightly greased pan. Flip it and butter the pan to baste the fish for a minute or so (rare inside).

Meal Prep Tips:

1. Store the pesto in the fridge.
2. When the salmon is done, cool entirely. Store in the fridge overnight or freeze for later.
3. When ready to eat, just serve over some lettuce with a dollop of pesto, slivered almonds, and shallots.

Creamy Salmon & Pasta

Serving Yields: 2

Macros: 3 g Net Carbs | 470 Calories | 21 g Protein |42 g Total Fats

Fixings Needed:

- Coconut oil – 2 tbsp.
- Zucchinis - 2
- Smoked salmon – 8 oz.
- Mayo – keto-friendly - .25 cup

How to Prepare:

1. Use a peeler or spiralizer to make noodle-like strands from the zucchini.
2. Warm up the oil over the med-high temperature setting. When hot, add the salmon and saute 2-3 minutes until golden brown.

3. Stir in the noodles and saute 1-2 more minutes.

Meal Prep Tips:

1. Store the noodles in the fridge after cooled overnight.
2. When it's time to eat, just stir in the mayo and divide the pasta between two dishes.
3. Serve and enjoy!

Chapter 7:

<u>Dinner Favorites</u>

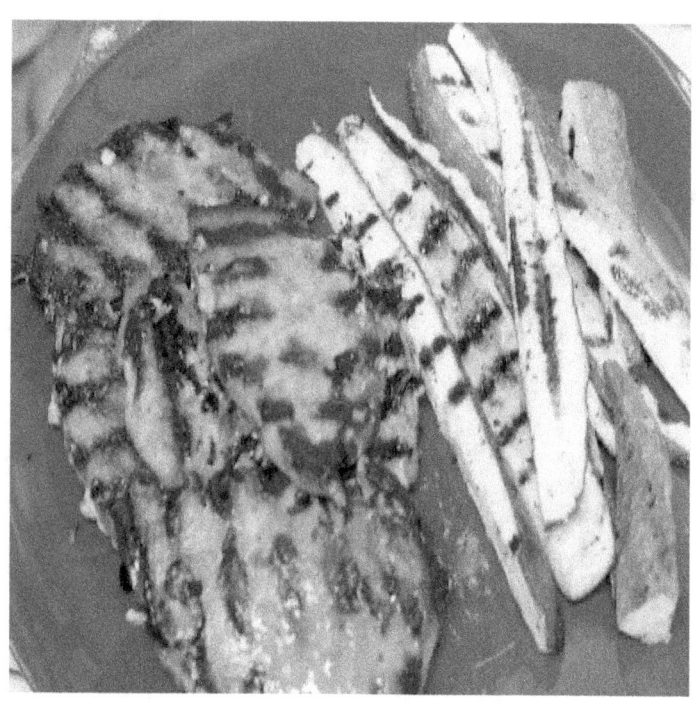

Beef Choices

Balsamic Beef Pot Roast

Serving Yields: 10

Macros: 3 g Net Carbs |393 Calories|30 g Protein |28 g Total Fats

Fixings Needed:

- Ground black pepper – 1 tsp.
- Kosher salt – 1 tbsp.
- Garlic powder – 1 tsp.
- Boneless chuck roast – 3 lb.
- Balsamic vinegar - .25 cup
- Chopped onion - .5 cup
- Water – 2 cups
- Xanthan gum - .25 tsp.
- For the Garnish: Chopped fresh parsley

How to Prepare:

1. Slice the roast in half and season with the garlic powder, pepper, and salt.
2. Prepare the pot using the saute function and brown the meat.
3. Pour in the onion, water, and vinegar. Secure the lid and set for 35 minutes. Natural release the pressure in the Instant Pot.
4. Add the meat to a container and break it apart. Discard fat and use the saute function to simmer the juices in the pot. Add the beef back after whisking in the xanthan gum. Gently stir and turn off the heat.

Meal Prep Tips:

1. Let the roast cool completely.
2. Store it in a heavy-duty freezer bag.
3. Thaw and warm it up. Garnish as desired.

Cumin Spiced Beef Wraps

Serving Yields: 2

Macros: 4 g Net Carbs | 375 Calories | 30 g Protein | 26 g Total Fats

Fixings Needed:

- Coconut oil – 1-2 tbsp.
- Diced onion – .25 of 1
- Ground beef - .66 lb.
- Chopped cilantro – 2 tbsp.
- Red bell pepper – 1 diced
- Minced ginger – 1 tsp.
- Cumin – 2 tsp.
- Minced garlic cloves – 4
- Pepper and salt - to taste
- Large cabbage leaves - 8

How to Prepare:

1. Warm up a frying pan and pour in the oil.
2. Saute the peppers, onions, and ground beef using medium heat.
3. When done, add the pepper, salt, cumin, ginger, cilantro, and garlic.

Meal Prep Tips:

1. Cool the burger entirely and add to storage containers.

Time to Eat:

2. Prepare the Leaves: Fill a large pot with water (3/4 full) and wait for it to boil. Cook each leaf for 20 seconds, plunge it in cold water and drain before placing it on your serving dish.
3. Reheat the beef mixture.
4. Scoop the mixture onto each leaf, fold, and enjoy.

Sweet and Sour Meatballs

Serving Yields: 5

Macros: 5 g Net Carbs | 295 Calories | 28 g Protein | 18.7 g Total Fats

Fixings Needed:

- Large egg - 1
- Ground beef – 1 lb.
- Onion powder - .5 tsp.
- Parmesan cheese - .25 cup

Fixings Needed for the Sauce:

- Soy sauce – 3 tbsp.
- Water – 1.5 cups
- Apple cider vinegar - .25 cup
- Erythritol – 1 cup
- Sugar-free ketchup - .33 cup
- Xanthan gum - .5 tsp.

How to Prepare:

1. Use your hands to combine the egg, beef, onion powder, and parmesan cheese in a mixing container. Shape the mixture into about thirty balls.

2. Add the meatballs to a heated saucepan and brown. Set them aside.

3. Pour in the soy sauce, water, vinegar, Erythritol, and ketchup using the same pan and stir.

4. Slowly, pour in the xanthan gum, but be sure to wait a couple of minutes in between pouring to be sure it thickens. Lower the temperature to low and simmer. Check the sauce every two minutes until it reaches the desired texture.

Meal Prep Tips:

1. You can add the sauce into the meatballs if you will be using the recipe within a day or so.
2. Or just simmer the sauce. Store the sauce and meatballs individually. Portion into 5 individual containers.
3. When ready to eat, just add the meatballs and sauce into a pan. Simmer for ten minutes on low.

Tasty Short Ribs

Serving Yields: 4

Macros: 2.5 g Net Carbs | 685 Calories | 25.7 g Protein |62 g Total Fats

Fixings Needed:

- Keto-friendly soy sauce - .25 cup
- Beef short ribs – 6 – 4 oz. each
- Rice vinegar – 2 tbsp.
- Fish sauce – 2 tbsp.
- Red pepper flakes - .5 tsp.
- Sesame seeds - .5 tsp.
- Onion powder - .5 tsp.
- Minced garlic - .5 tsp.
- Ground ginger – 1 tsp.
- Salt – 1 tbsp.
- Cardamom - .25 tsp.

How to Prepare:

1. Mix the fish sauce, vinegar, and alternative soy sauce.
2. Arrange the ribs in a dish with high sides. Add the sauce and marinate for up to 1 hour.
3. Combine all of the spices together. Take the ribs from the dish and sprinkle with the rub.
4. Warm up the grill (med-high) and cook for 3 to 5 minutes on each side.

Meal Prep Tips:

1. Put the ribs in a platter to cool.
2. Place in freezer bags or into plastic containers (4 portions) until it's time to serve and enjoy.

Chicken Choices

Authentic Butter Chicken

Serving Yields: 6

Macros: 6 g Net Carbs | 293 Calories | 25 g Protein | 17 g Total Fats

Fixings Needed:

- Chicken breast – 1.5 lb.
- Garam masala – 2 tbsp.
- Grated fresh ginger – 3 tsp.
- Minced garlic – 3 tsp.
- Plain yogurt – 4 oz.
- Coconut oil - 1 tbsp.

Fixings Needed for the Sauce:

- Ghee or butter – 2 tbsp.
- Onion - 1
- Fresh ginger - grated – 2 tsp.

- Minced garlic – 2 tsp.

- Crushed tomatoes - 14.5 oz.

- Ground coriander – 1 tbsp.

- Garam masala - .5 tbsp.

- Chilli powder – 1 tsp.

- Cumin – 2 tsp.

- Heavy cream - .5 cup

- Salt – to your liking

Optional Toppings:

- Cilantro
- Cauliflower rice

How to Prepare:

1. In a large dish, use a sharp knife and dice the chicken breasts into 2-inch pieces. Stir in 2 tablespoons garam masala, 1 teaspoon grated ginger, and 1 teaspoon minced garlic. Add in the yogurt, stir to combine. Chill at least 30 minutes.

2. For the Sauce: Place the onion, ginger, garlic, crushed tomatoes, and spices in a blender. Pulse until creamy smooth. Place the sauce to the side for now.

3. Warm up the oil in a good-sized pan using the medium-high heat setting. Arrange the chicken in the skillet, browning 3 to 4 minutes per side. Once browned, pour in the sauce, cook 5 to 6 minutes longer.

4. Stir in the heavy cream and ghee, continue to cook another minute. Taste

for salt and add additional if needed. Top with cilantro and serve with cauliflower rice if desired.

5. Note: Nutritional information does not include cauliflower rice.

Meal Prep Tips:

1. Prepare the chicken and place into the storage container of choice. Store in the fridge or freezer – with the container clearly marked.

2. Prepare the sauce and place in baggies unless you are planning on using quickly. If you are serving within several days, just prepare and store it in an airtight container.

3. When ready to prepare, just continue with step 4, combining the cream and ghee with the chicken, etc.

Buffalo Chicken Burgers

Serving Yields: 2 burgers

Macros: 1 g Net Carbs | 488 Calories | 43 g Protein | 34 g Total Fats

Fixings Needed:

- Chicken breasts – 8 oz. cooked
- Room-temperature cream cheese - 2 oz.
- Shredded mozzarella cheese - .5 cup
- Frank's Red-Hot Sauce or your choice – 2 tbsp.
- Coconut oil or ghee for frying

How to Prepare:

1. Either chop or shred the prepared chicken and combine with the rest of the fixings.

2. Place the fixings in the microwave for 15 to 20 seconds to help compact the ingredients. Form two medium patties and place on a plate. Store in the freezer for about 15 minutes.

3. Warm up a skillet using the high heat setting. Add the fat and patties. Prepare the burgers for 2 to 3 minutes per side.

4. Serve when crispy brown.

Meal Prep Tips:

1. Prepare the chicken and mix to form patties.

2. Freeze or cook and freeze the patties.

Chicken and Asparagus Pan Dinner

Serving Yields: 8

Macros: 4 g Net Carbs | 439 Calories | 63 g Protein | 18.2 g Total Fats

Fixings Needed:

- Chicken breasts – 4 lbs.
- Avocado oil – 1 tbsp.
- Trimmed asparagus – 1 lb.
- Sun-dried tomatoes - 4
- Thick-cut bacon – 4 slices
- Salt – 1 tsp.
- Pepper - .25 tsp.
- Provolone cheese – 8 slices
- Also Needed: 1 baking pan

How to Prepare:

1. Slice the chicken into 8 thin pieces. Chop the bacon and tomatoes into one-inch pieces.

2. Warm up the oven temperature to 400°F.

3. Add the oil to the baking pan along with the chicken and asparagus. Top it off with the tomatoes and bacon. Sprinkle some pepper and salt for seasoning.

4. Bake until the chicken reaches 160°F internally or about 25 minutes.

5. Toss in the asparagus and cheese.

6. Garnish with some bacon and tomatoes. Bake another three to four minutes until the cheese has melted.

Meal Prep Tips:

1. Simply prepare the chicken and store in the fridge for several days.
2. Place into plastic bins or freezer bags until ready to use.
3. Prepare the asparagus when ready to eat and combine with the cheese. Garnish and serve.

Chicken & Bacon Patties

Serving Yields: 10 Patties

Macros: 1.5 g Net Carbs | 95.6 Calories | 7.25 g Protein | 6.16 g Total Fats

Fixings Needed:

- Bacon – 4 slices
- Chicken breast – 1 can – 12 oz.
- Medium bell peppers - 2
- Large egg - 1
- Sun-dried tomato pesto - .25 cup
- Parmesan cheese - .25 cup
- Coconut flour – 3 tbsp.

How to Prepare:

1. In the food processor, finely chop the peppers and add them to a mixing container. Use a paper towel to pat the excess liquid from the veggies after mixing.

2. Prepare the bacon – cook until crispy. Cool and chop it with the chicken. Add it to the processor until almost smooth. Combine all of the fixings and make patties.

3. Fry on the med-hi to the medium setting in a skillet with a little oil.

4. Once browned on one side, flip it and continue cooking until done. Let the grease drain on the towels.

Meal Prep Tips:

1. Let them cool completely. Store in the fridge for a day or so.
2. Store in freezer bags and place in the freezer for later. Be sure to mark its contents clearly.
3. When it is time to eat, just garnish with your favorite toppings but remember to count the extras.

Chicken & Gravy

Serving Yields: 2

Macros: 4 g Net Carbs | 375 Calories | 30 g Protein | 26 g Total Fats

Fixings Needed:

- Coconut oil – 1-2 tbsp.
- Diced onion – .25 of 1
- Ground beef - .66 lb.
- Chopped cilantro – 2 tbsp.
- Red bell pepper – 1 diced
- Minced ginger – 1 tsp.
- Cumin – 2 tsp.
- Minced garlic cloves – 4
- Pepper and salt - to taste
- Large cabbage leaves - 8

How to Prepare:

1. Warm up a frying pan and pour in the oil.
2. Saute the peppers, onions, and ground beef using medium heat.
3. When done, add the pepper, salt, cumin, ginger, cilantro, and garlic.

Meal Prep Tips:

1. Cool the burger entirely and add to storage containers.

Time to Eat:

2. Prepare the Leaves: Fill a large pot with water (3/4 full) and wait for it to boil. Cook each leaf for 20 seconds, plunge it

in cold water and drain before placing it on your serving dish.

3. Reheat the beef mixture.

4. Scoop the mixture onto each leaf, fold, and enjoy.

Chicken Kiev

Serving Yields: 2

Macros: 4 g Net Carbs | 510 Calories|50 g Protein |33 g Total Fats

Fixings Needed:

- Breasts of chicken – 2 – 6 oz. each
- Cloves of garlic - 2
- Butter – 4 tbsp.
- Green onion – 1 stalk
- Parsley - pinch
- Tarragon - pinch
- Pepper and salt – to taste
- Pork rinds – 1 oz.
- Coconut flour - .25 cup
- Egg - 1

How to Prepare:

1. Set the oven temperature to 350°F.

2. Use a tenderizing hammer to pound the chicken until they are approximately one-half-inch to one-inch thick. Flavor it with the tarragon, pepper, salt, and parsley.

3. Add chopped bits of butter, garlic, and green onion evenly to the pieces of chicken. Close with toothpicks.

4. Crush the pork rinds for the crumbs (NutriBullet for a few seconds works great.)

5. Make dredging dishes, one each for flour, a beaten egg, and the pork rind crumbs.

6. Cover the chicken with the flour, egg, then the rinds. Close them tightly with a toothpick. Let the fixings chill in the fridge for about ½ hour.

7. Fry the breasts until browned on all sides in a lightly oiled pan.
8. Transfer and arrange them in a baking dish.
9. Bake for approximately 20 minutes. Baste with any leftover butter.

Meal Prep Tips:

1. Let the chicken cool completely. Store in the fridge for one to two days.
2. You can also portion the fixings into freezer bags and store for later.
3. When ready to serve, add to a bed of lettuce.

Chicken Parmesan

Serving Yields: 2

Macros: 3 g Net Carbs | 600 Calories | 74 g Protein | 32 g Total Fats

Fixings Needed:

- Breasts of chicken – 1 lb.
- Parmesan cheese – 2 tbsp.
- Pork rinds – 1 oz.
- Egg – 1
- Marinara sauce - .5 cup
- Shredded mozzarella - .5 cup

Possible Garnish Ingredients:

- Garlic powder
- Oregano
- Freshly cracked black pepper
- Salt

How to Prepare:

1. Program the oven temperature to 350°F.
2. Use a food processor/Magic Bullet to crush the pork rinds and parmesan cheese. Add them to a bowl.
3. Pound the chicken breasts until they are ½-inch thick. Beat the egg and dip the chicken in for an egg wash. Dip the chicken into the crumbs.
4. Arrange the breasts on a baking sheet that is lightly greased. Sprinkle with the seasonings and bake for 25 minutes.

Meal Prep Tips:

1. When done, just cool the prepared chicken. Store in the fridge for a day or so. After that time, add to a freezer bag or storage container awaiting a side dish.

2. Time to Serve: Pour the marinara sauce over each portion. Garnish with the mozzarella and bake for 15 minutes.

3. Enjoy with spinach.

Pork Choices

Asian-Inspired Pork Chops

Serving Yields: 4

Macros: 3 g Net Carbs | 327.4 Calories| 41.3 g Protein | 15.6 g Total Fats

Fixings Needed:

- Pork chops – boneless -4
- Cloves of garlic – 4 halved
- Lemongrass – peeled and diced – 1 stalk
- Star anise – 1 medium
- Almond flour – 1 tbsp.
- Fish sauce – 1 tbsp.
- Sambal chili paste - .5 tbsp.
- Sugar-free ketchup - .5 tbsp.
- Soy sauce – 1.5 tsp.
- Sesame oil – 1 tsp.

- Peppercorns - .5 tsp.
- Five Spice - .5 tsp.

How to Prepare:

1. Pound the chops until they are about ½ - inch thick.
2. Slice the garlic into halves. Grind the star anise and peppercorns with a pestle and mortar or in a blender. Toss in the garlic and lemongrass. Mix until pureed and add the soy sauce, five spice powder, sesame oil, and fish sauce. Stir well.
3. Place the chops in a baking pan, add the marinade, and coat well. Cover for one to two hours at room temperature.

4. Lightly coat the chops with the flour and add to a pan set on the high-heat setting. Sear about two minutes on each side. Place on the cutting board and chop into several strips.
5. Make a sauce by combining the ketchup and chili paste. Yummy!

Meal Prep Tips:

1. Prepare the chops and place into containers or freezer bags or store in the fridge or freezer – your choice.
2. Prepare the sauce on the day you are ready to serve or store it in 4 individual containers for added convenience.

Chicken Fried Pork Chops

Serving Yields: 4

Macros: 0.8 g Net Carbs |390 Calories| 28.8 g Protein |20.8 g Total Fats

Fixings Needed:

- Bone-out pork chops – 4 medium - 16 oz. ea.
- Ground pork rinds – 1 oz.
- Chopped nuts – 1 tbsp.
- Flaxseed meal – 2 tbsp.
- Salt – 1 tsp.
- Almond flour – 2 tbsp.
- Large egg - 1
- Oil or fat of choice – 4 tbsp.

How to Prepare:

1. In a food processor, grind the rinds to a powder and combine with the flaxseed meal, flour, and nut blend.
2. Warm up the oil/fat in a skillet using the med-hi setting.
3. Whisk an egg in a dish and dip the chop. Dip in the rind mixture (step 1). Coat well and fry for about four to five minutes for each side. The internal temperature should reach 145°F.
4. Serve and enjoy!

Meal Prep Tips:

1. This one is easy for meal prep. All you need to do is prepare the chops and store in the freezer bag or in the fridge for tomorrow — your choice.

Pan-Fried Pork Chops

Serving Yields: 3

Macros: 4 g Net Carbs | 385 Calories | 22.1 g Protein | 27 g Total Fats

Fixings Needed:

- Coconut flour - .5 cup
- Salt and black pepper – 1 tsp. each
- Pork chops - 3
- Butter – 1 tbsp.

How to Prepare:

Combine all of the dry fixings in a large mixing container.

Pat the chops dry with a paper towel.

Melt the butter in a skillet on the stovetop.

Cover the chops with the mixture and prepare each side for 4 to 5 minutes.

Serve with your favorite side dishes.

Meal Prep Tips:

1. Once the chops have finished cooking. Let them cool completely.
2. Place them in an air-tight container and use within a couple of days.
3. You can also place them individually in freezer bags for later. Be sure to date and mark the preparation method.

Parmesan Crusted Pork Chops

Serving Yields: 14

Macros: 3 g Net Carbs | 354 Calories | 33 g Protein | 34 g Total Fats

Fixings Needed:

- Parmesan cheese – 6 oz.
- Pork chops - 14
- Large eggs - 2
- Almond flour - .75 cup
- Pepper and salt – to your liking
- For Frying: Bacon grease

How to Prepare:

1. Heat up the oven to 400°F.
2. Grate the parmesan and mix with the flour and spices.

3. Whisk the eggs in a shallow dish.

4. Dip the chops in the eggs, then the parmesan mixture.

5. Fry in the bacon grease on each side for one minute.

6. Arrange on a baking dish in the oven, bake until done.

Meal Prep Tips:

1. Store safely in the fridge for several days.

2. Place in freezer bags and store. Make sure you date and add the name of the recipe to recall it later.

Pulled Pork

Serving Yields: 8

Macros: 2.2 g Net Carbs |464 Calories| 43 g Protein | 30.2 g Total Fats

Fixings Needed:

- Boneless pork shoulder – 3 lb.
- Chopped white onion - 1
- Bay leaves - 3
- Smoked paprika – 1 tsp.
- Pink Himalayan salt – 3 tsp.
- Garlic powder – 2 tsp.

How to Prepare:

1. Heat up the slow cooker using the low setting. Combine the paprika, salt, and garlic powder. Slice the pork into chunks and rub into the spices.

2. Chop the onion and toss it into the cooker along with the pork. Add the bay leaves and close the lid. Cook for 10 hours on low.
3. When ready, shred and let cool.

Meal Prep Tips:

1. Add the shredded pork to individual bags for the freezer or into compartmentalized dishes to await a veggie.
2. Be sure to date the containers and label with the name of its content.

Chapter 8:

<u>Sides - Snacks &</u>

<u>Appetizers</u>

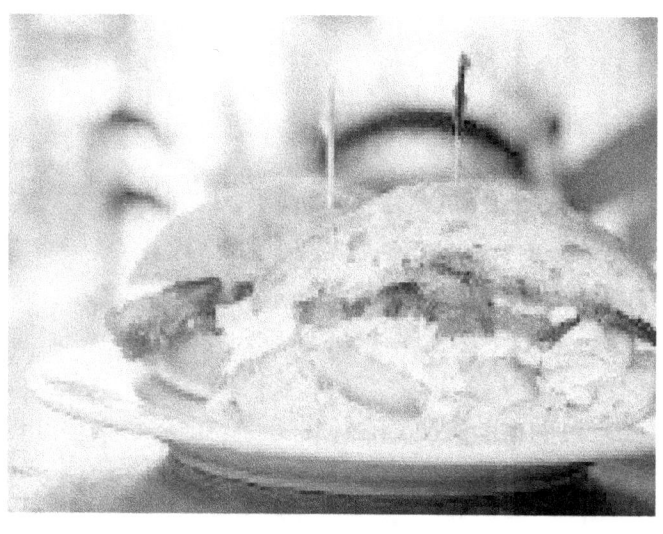

For most of the side veggie dishes, it is usually best to prepare no more than 24 hours ahead of time (unless otherwise noted in the recipe). You can use these delicious sides any time.

Sides

Asparagus & Garlic

Serving Yields: 4

Macros: 2 g Net Carbs | 61 Calories | 1 g Protein | 6 g Total Fats

Fixings Needed:

- Minced garlic – 1 tbsp.
- Fresh asparagus – 1 bunch
- Butter – 2 tbsp.

How to Prepare:

1. Rinse the asparagus and separate each of the stalks. Boil them for 2-3 minutes. Drain and chill in a dish of cold water.
2. Warm up the garlic and butter in a skillet. Fry the asparagus with them until browned.

Meal Prep Tips:

1. Once they are cooled, you can store them in one dish.
2. You can also divide them into individual containers with other choices for later.

Baked Radishes & Brown Butter Sauce

Serving Yields: 2

Macros: 2 g Net Carbs | 181 Calories | 1 g Protein | 19 g Total Fats

Fixings Needed:

- Olive oil – 1 tbsp.
- Halved radishes – 2 cups
- Butter – 2 tbsp.
- Freshly ground black pepper & Pink Himalayan salt – to taste
- Freshly chopped flat-leaf Italian parsley – 1 tbsp.

How to Prepare:

1. arm up the oven to reach 450°F.

2. Cut the radishes into halves and toss into the oil. Sprinkle with the pepper and salt. Spread them on a baking sheet – single layered. Bake for 15 minutes. Stir about halfway through the cycle.

3. After they have roasted 10 minutes, use the medium heat setting on the stovetop to melt the butter mixed with the salt. Simmer until it's a nutty brown (3 min.). Pour the butter into a mug and set aside.

Meal Prep Tips:

1. Let everything cool completely. Take the radishes out of the oven and portion into two plates.
2. You can divide the butter into two containers or leave in one container for a day or two.
3. When ready to serve. Heat up and add the butter and top it off with the fresh parsley.

Buffalo Cauliflower Bites

Serving Yields: 4

Macros: 3 g Net Carbs | 130 Calories | 2 g Protein | 12 g Total Fats

Fixings Needed:

- Cauliflower florets – 4 cups
- Cracked black pepper – to taste
- Sea salt - .25 tsp.
- Cayenne pepper - .25 tsp.
- Salted butter – 4 tbsp.
- Hot sauce - .25 cup
- Minced garlic – 1 clove
- Paprika - .25 tsp
- Optional – Blue cheese dressing

How to Prepare:

1. Warm up the oven until it reaches 375°F.
2. Arrange the florets on a paper-lined baking tray.
3. Whisk the cayenne, black pepper, salt, paprika, garlic, butter, and hot sauce. Pour into a microwavable-safe dish for 30 seconds or until smooth.
4. Empty the sauce over the florets in the pan and bake for 25 minutes.

Meal Prep Tips:

1. Cool thoroughly. Add to individual containers or freezer bags.
2. You can store in the fridge for a couple of days.
3. Serve with a bowl of blue cheese dressing for dipping.

Caprese Salad

Serving Yields: 4

Macros: 5 g Net Carbs | 191 Calories | 7.7 g Protein | 63.5 g Total Fats

Fixings Needed:

- Grape tomatoes – 3 cups
- Peeled garlic cloves - 4
- Avocado oil – 2 tbsp.
- Mozzarella balls – 19 pearl-sized
- Baby spinach leaves – 4 cups
- Fresh basil leaves - .25 cup
- Brine reserved from the cheese – 1 tbsp.
- Pesto - 1 tbsp.

How to Prepare:

1. Use a sheet of aluminum foil to cover a baking tray.
2. Set the oven temperature setting to 400°F.
3. Arrange the cloves and tomatoes on the baking pan and drizzle with the oil. Bake for 20-30 minutes until the tops are slightly browned.
4. Drain the liquid (saving one tablespoon) from the mozzarella. Mix the pesto with the brine.
5. Arrange the spinach in a large serving bowl. Transfer the tomatoes to the dish along with the roasted garlic.

Meal Prep Tips:

- Cool the ingredients thoroughly. Place in closed containers until time to use.
- Drizzle with the pesto sauce. Garnish with the mozzarella balls and freshly torn basil leaves.

Cauliflower Mac & Cheese

Serving Yields: 4

Macros: 7 g Net Carbs | 294 Calories | 11 g Protein | 23 g Total Fats

Fixings Needed:

- Butter – 3 tbsp.
- Cauliflower – 1 head
- Cheddar cheese – 1 cup
- Black pepper & sea salt - to taste
- Unsweetened almond milk - .25 cup
- Heavy cream - .25 cup

How to Prepare:

1. Slice the cauliflower into small florets and shred the cheese.

2. Heat up the oven to reach 450ºF. Use a piece of aluminum foil or parchment paper to line a baking sheet.
3. Melt 2 tbsp. of butter. Toss the florets and butter. Give it a shake of pepper and salt. Place the cauliflower on the baking pan and roast 10-15 minutes.
4. Warm up the rest of the butter, milk, heavy cream, and cheese in the microwave or double boiler.
5. Pour on the cheese.

Meal Prep Tips:

1. Prepare the mac and cheese and let it cool thoroughly.
2. Store in an airtight container to use within a day or so.
3. Warm up and serve.

Cobb Salad

Serving Yields: 2

Macros: 3 g Net Carbs | 600 Calories| 43 g Protein | 48 g Total Fats

Fixings Needed:

- Hard-boiled egg - 1
- Spinach – 1 cup
- Bacon strips - 2
- Campari tomato - .5 of 1
- Chicken breast – 2 oz.
- Avocado - .25 of 1
- Olive oil – 1 tbsp.
- White vinegar - .5 tsp.

How to Prepare:

1. Prepare the bacon and chicken shred or slice the chicken.
2. Cut all of the ingredients into small pieces. Toss them to a bowl.

Meal Prep Tips:

1. You can add the prepared salad into individual bowls and securely close with a lid.
2. When it is time to eat, drizzle with the vinegar and oil.
3. Toss gently and serve.

Hibachi Mushrooms – Japanese Style

Serving Yields: 4

Macros: 3 g Net Carbs |102 Calories| 3.4 g Protein | 8.9 g Total Fats

Fixings Needed:

- Unsalted butter – 3 tbsp.
- White onion, diced - .5 of 1
- Button mushrooms, halved or quartered – 8 oz.
- Tamari – 3 tbsp.
- Pepper – 0.125 tsp.
- Salt – to your liking

How to Prepare:

1. Heat the butter over medium-high heat in a 10.5" cast iron skillet.
2. Stir in onion and mushrooms. Saute for about 5 minutes then add in tamari, continue to cook until the sauce has almost evaporated.

Meal Prep Tips:

1. Season with salt to taste. Let them cool completely.
2. You can portion them into a freezer baggie or plastic container for freezer storage. Be sure to remove the air from the chosen container.
3. You can also place them in the fridge in a closed container to use within a day or so.

Lemony Green Beans with Almonds

Serving Yields: 4

Macros: 6.5 g Net Carbs |131 Calories| 3.5 g Protein | 9.8 g Total Fats

Fixings Needed:

- Lemon juice – 1-2 tbsp.
- Unrefined sea salt - .5 tsp
- Garlic cloves - 4
- Fresh green beans – 1 lb.
- Sliced organic almonds - .33 cup
- Olive oil– 2 tbsp.

How to Prepare:

1. Trim the beans and steam until tender and crispy. Add the salt and lemon juice - toss gently.

2. Warm up the olive oil in a pan using the med-low setting. Blend in the almonds and cook until the almonds start changing colors and add the garlic. Continue cooking for 30 seconds. Cook the garlic no more than 60 seconds because it will lose its nutrients.
3. Mix everything together and toss well.

Meal Prep Tips:

1. Prepare the recipe. Let it cool completely.
2. If you have a container system for your prep, add it to another dish.
3. You can also store it in an individual container for the freezer or in a regular dish for serving in the next day or so.

Snack Choices

Healthy Chia Bars

Serving Yields: 14

Macros: 1.5 g Net Carbs | 121 Calories| 2.5 g Protein | 11 g Total Fats

Fixings Needed:

- Toasted almonds - .5 cup
- Coconut oil – divided – 1 tbsp. (+) 1 tsp.
- Erythritol – 4 tbsp. - divided
- Butter - 2 tbsp.
- Heavy cream - .25 tsp.
- Liquid stevia - .25 tsp.
- Vanilla extract – 1.5 tsp.
- Unsweetened & shredded coconut flakes - .5 cup
- Chia seeds - .25 cup
- Coconut cream - .5 cup

- Coconut flour – 2 tbsp.
- Also Needed: Food Processor

How to Prepare:

1. Add the toasted almonds into the food processor and pulse until crumbly.
2. Toss in 1 tablespoon of the coconut oil and 2 tablespoons of the erythritol. Continue processing until you have almond butter. (Now you have another new usable product.)
3. Warm up a pan and add the butter, heavy cream, erythritol, stevia, and vanilla. Stir until they're bubbly and fold in the almond butter. Stir to blend.
4. In a blender, grind the chia seeds to make a powdery mix. In another pan, toast the coconut flakes and mix with the chia seeds. Melt the coconut cream in a separate skillet.

5. Now, combine all of the fixings and add the melted coconut cream, flour, and coconut oil. Store in the fridge for one hour.

Meal Prep Tips:

1. When it's ready, slice into squares and store in the refrigerator.
2. For convenience, you can place them into individual dishes or freezer bags.

Peanut Butter Protein Bars

Serving Yields: 12 Bars

Macros: 3 g Net Carbs |172 Calories| 7 g Protein | 14 g Total Fats

Fixings Needed:

- Keto-friendly chunky peanut butter – 1 cup
- Egg whites - 2
- Almonds - .5 cup
- Cashews - .5 cup
- Almond meal – 1.5 cups

How to Prepare:

1. Warm up the oven ahead of time to 350°F.
2. Combine all of the fixings and add to the prepared dish.
3. Bake for 15 minutes and cut into 12 pieces once they're cooled.

Meal Prep Tips:

1. Store in the fridge to keep them fresh.

Fat Bombs

Almond Butter Fat Bombs

Serving Yields: 8

Macros: 1.7 g Net Carbs | 145 Calories|1.5 g Protein | 14.7 g Total Fats

Fixings Needed:

- Almond butter – 9.5 tbsp.
- Melted coconut oil - .75 cup
- Liquid stevia – .25 tsp. or to your taste
- Melted salted butter – 9 tbsp.
- Cocoa – 3 tbsp.

How to Prepare:

2. Combine all of the components listed until smooth.
3. Add the final product to 24 mini muffin molds or use silicone candy molds.

Meal Prep Tips:

1. Freeze for a minimum of 30 minutes or until frozen solid for prep.
2. Pop them out and enjoy. Store in the freezer in an airtight container or zipper freezer baggie.

Blueberry Cream Cheese Fat Bombs

Serving Yields: 12

Macros: 1 g Net Carbs |67 Calories| 0.96 g Protein | 7.4 g Total Fats

Fixings Needed:

- Cream cheese – 1.5 cups
- Fresh or frozen berries – 1 cup
- Swerve – 2-3 tbsp.
- Vanilla extract – 1 tbsp.
- Coconut oil - .5 cup

How to Prepare:

1. For 30 to 60 minutes before preparation time, place the cream cheese on the countertop to become room temperature.
2. Take the stems off the berries and rinse. Pour into a blender. Mix well until smooth.
3. Pour in the Swerve and extract. Blend in the oil and cream cheese.
4. Add the mixture to candy molds and freeze for approximately two hours.

Meal Prep Tips:

1. Once the bombs are solid, just pop them out.
2. Store in freezer bags or another safe freezer container.

Chocolate Fat Bombs

Serving Yields: 24

Macros: 1 g Net Carbs | 180 Calories|3 g Protein | 21 g Total Fats

Fixings Needed:

- Coconut oil - .5 cup
- Splenda or your preference – 3 packets
- Walnut or almond butter - .25 cup
- Sugar-free coffee liqueur syrup – ex. Da Vinci – 2 tbsp.
- Heavy whipping cream - .25 cup
- Walnut halves - 24
- Also Needed: Silicon molds

How to Prepare:

1. Use a glass measuring cup and add the oil, walnut butter, coffee liqueur, cocoa powder, and sweetener.
2. Microwave for 30-40 seconds. Stir the contents until the oil melts.
3. Stir in the cream and pour into the molds. Arrange a nut in each one.

Meal Prep Tips:

1. Freeze the bombs until solid.
2. Leave them in the molds or pop them out and add them to a storage or container.
3. If you are planning a trip, add a bunch to individual serving bags for a quick snack.

Coffee Fat Bombs

Serving Yields: 15

Macros: -0- g Net Carbs | 45 Calories| -0- g Protein | 4 g Total Fats

Fixings Needed:

- Cream cheese – room temperature – 4.4 oz.
- Powdered Xylitol – 2 tbsp.
- Instant coffee – 1 tbsp.
- Coconut oil – 1 tbsp.
- Unsweetened cocoa powder – 1 tbsp.
- Room temperature butter – 1 tbsp.

How to Prepare:

1. Take the butter and cream cheese out of the fridge about an hour before it's time to begin.
2. With a blender/food processor, blitz the xylitol and coffee into a fine powder. Add the hot water to form a pasty mix.
3. Blend in the butter, cream cheese, cocoa powder, and coconut oil.
4. Add to ice cube trays and freeze a minimum of one to two hours.

Meal Prep Tips:

1. Use Ziplock bags to keep them fresh in the freezer.

Lemonade Fat Bombs

Serving Yields: 2

Macros: 7 g Net Carbs | 404 Calories| 4 g Protein | 43 g Total Fats

Fixings Needed:

- Cream cheese – 4 oz.
- Butter – 2 oz.
- Lemon zest & juice - .5 of 1 lemon
- Swerve - 2 tsp.
- Pink Himalayan salt – 1 pinch or to taste

How to Prepare:

2. Take the butter and cream cheese out of the fridge and let it become room temperature before using. Zest the lemon and juice it into a small dish.

3. In another container, mix the butter with the cream cheese. Use a hand mixer to combine all of the fixings until well mixed.

4. Spoon the mixture into small molds or cupcake paper liners in a muffin tin pan.

5. Stick the chosen holder in the freezer for two hours.

Meal Prep Tips:

1. Take them out of the molds and put them in a zipper-top baggie to enjoy any time.

2. Store in the freezer for up to three months.

Appetizers

Chicken Salad Deviled Eggs

Serving Yields: 6

Macros: 2 g Net Carbs | 128 Calories| 13 g Protein | 7 g Total Fats

Fixings Needed:

- Old Bay Seasoning – 1 dash
- Lemon pepper – .5 tsp.
- Dill - .5 tsp.
- Celery salt – 1 pinch
- Chopped onion – 1 tbsp.
- Dijon mustard – 1 tsp.
- Mayonnaise – 2 tbsp.
- Shredded chicken – 1 cup
- Large eggs – 6

How to Prepare:

1. Combine all of the fixings, omit the eggs, and store in the fridge for later.
2. Gently place the eggs in a pot of water (just enough to cover the eggs).
3. Set the temperature on high until it boils and lower the setting to medium.
4. Boil for 15 minutes and transfer to cool under cold running water.
5. Remove the shell and slice the eggs into halves. Remove the yolk and fill with the salad mixture. Sprinkle with the old bay seasoning.
6. Note: Discard the yolks or use in another recipe. Total time is just 30 minutes.

Meal Prep Tips:

1. These eggs are a great solution for those times when you want to entertain your guests or just want a goodie to add to your dinner tray.
2. Just make a batch and see how quickly they disappear.

Little Smokies

Serving Yields: 12

Macros: 3.3 g Net Carbs |177 Calories| 7.3 g Protein | 15.1 g Total Fats

Fixings Needed:

- Cocktail Smokies – 24 oz.
- Avocado oil – 2 tbsp.
- Fixings Needed for the BBQ Sauce:
- Unsweetened ketchup – 1 cup
- Water - .5 cup
- Apple cider vinegar – 3 tbsp.
- Brown swerve - .25 cup
- Worcestershire sauce – 1 tsp.
- Natural maple flavoring – 2 tsp.
- Dijon mustard – 1 tsp.
- Salt - .5 tsp.
- Garlic powder - .5 tsp
- Black pepper - .25 tsp.

- Onion powder - .5 tsp
- Also Needed: 1 iron skillet

How to Prepare:

1. Combine the sauce fixings in a jar or other container and set to the side for now.
2. Warm up the oil in the skillet using the med-high heat setting.
3. Sear the smokies for 2 to 3 minutes until they begin to change color.
4. Stir in the sauce and lower the heat to simmer for (10 to 15 min.) or until thickened to your liking.
5. Note: The average serving size is 6, but it will depend on the brand used. (Trader Joe's Cocktail Pups were used in this one.)

Meal Prep Tips:

1. This is a great choice to prep for a party. Just prepare a day or so before the party and you are ready to go!

2. Freeze if you want to save them for later. They should be good for up to one to two months. If they're constantly frozen at 0°F, they should last indefinitely.

Condiments – The Keto-Friendly Way

Condiments are the items that can cause issues with your new way of eating using keto techniques. Problems may arise of how to remain in ketosis and still enjoy the dining condiments that are offered in most supermarkets. The short answer is – you cannot. Are you wondering how to prepare that keto-friendly meal? The answer is simple. This segment is a special bonus for some of those times when nothing else will work in your favorite keto recipe. These are so delicious that you will not realize they are very healthy choices. Keep your ketosis in line with one of these favorites:

Keto-Friendly Dips & Sauces

For the easiest prep for your dips and sauces, just prepare each choice and store according to the recipe.

Lemon-Dill Tartar Sauce

Serving Yields: 1

Macros: 1 g Net Carbs |85 Calories| -0- g Protein | 9 g Total Fats

Fixings Needed:

- Mayonnaise – 1 cup
- Dill pickles – 2
- Dill pickle juice - 1 tbsp.
- Freshly squeezed lemon juice - .5 tsp.
- Sea salt – 1 pinch
- Onion powder - .5 tsp.
- Black pepper- to taste

How to Prepare:

1. Combine all of the fixings.
2. You can store the sauce in an air-tight container for up to three days.

Ketchup

Macros: 1.1 g Net Carbs |9 Calories| -0- g Protein | -0- g Total Fats

Fixings Needed:

- Diced tomatoes – 1 can organic – 14.5 oz. (+) 1 can water
- Italian seasoning – 1 tsp.
- Star anise – 1 piece
- White vinegar - .5 tbsp.
- Freshly ground pepper
- Salt
- Optional: Erythritol – to your liking

How to Prepare:

1. In a small saucepan, add the tomatoes and add a can of water.
2. Stir in the herbs and anise. Simmer using the low heat setting for one hour, stirring frequently.
3. Transfer the pan from the heat and add the vinegar. Add any other seasonings as desired and remove the star anise.
4. Let it cool and puree into a smooth ketchup sauce using a blender/food processor.

Meal Prep Tips:

1. Store in the fridge for no more than 4 days.

Mayonnaise

Avocado Mayo

Serving Yields: 4

Macros: 4 g Net Carbs | 1 g Protein | 5 g Total Fats

Fixings Needed:

- Avocado - .5 of 1 medium
- Pink salt – 1 pinch
- Ground cayenne pepper - .5 tsp.
- Lime juice - .5 of 1
- Olive oil - .25 cup

How to Prepare:

2. Dice the avocado and toss into a blender or food processor. Pulse and add in the salt, cayenne, cilantro, and lime juice.

3. When smooth, stir in the oil – 1 tbsp. at a time -

4. You can store the mayo for up to one week in a sealed glass bottle.

Sriracha Mayo

Serving Yields: 4

Macros: 2 g Net Carbs|1 g Protein | 22 g Total Fats

Fixings Needed:

- Sriracha sauce – 2 tbsp.
- Paprika - .25 tsp.
- Mayonnaise - .5 cup
- Onion - .5 tsp.
- Garlic - .5 tsp.

How to Prepare:

1. Whisk the fixings together in a small container.
2. It will store easily for up to one week in the fridge.

Salad Dressings

Blue Cheese Chunky Style Dressing

Serving Yields: 4

Macros: 3 g Net Carbs | 7 g Protein | 32 g Total Fats

Fixings Needed:

- Mayonnaise - .5 cup
- Sour cream - .5 cup
- Lemon juice - .5 of 1
- Worcestershire sauce - .5 tsp.
- Black pepper and salt – to your liking
- Crumbled blue cheese – 2 oz.

How to Prepare:

1. Whisk all of the fixings except for the cheese until well mixed.
2. Fold in the cheese gently and store in a closed glass dish for up to one week.

Caesar Dressing

Serving Yields: 4

Macros: 2 g Net Carbs |2 g Protein | 23 g Total Fats

Fixings Needed:

- Mayonnaise - .5 cup
- Dijon mustard – 1 tbsp.
- Lemon juice - .5 of 1
- Worcestershire sauce - .5 tsp.
- Parmesan cheese - .25 cup
- Freshly cracked black pepper – 1 pinch
- Pink Himalayan salt – to taste

How to Prepare:

1. Whisk the lemon juice, mustard, mayonnaise, salt, pepper, and Worcestershire sauce. Stir well and add the parmesan.
2. Whisk until smooth.
3. You can store up to one week in a glass container in the fridge.

Chapter 9:

<u>Desserts</u>

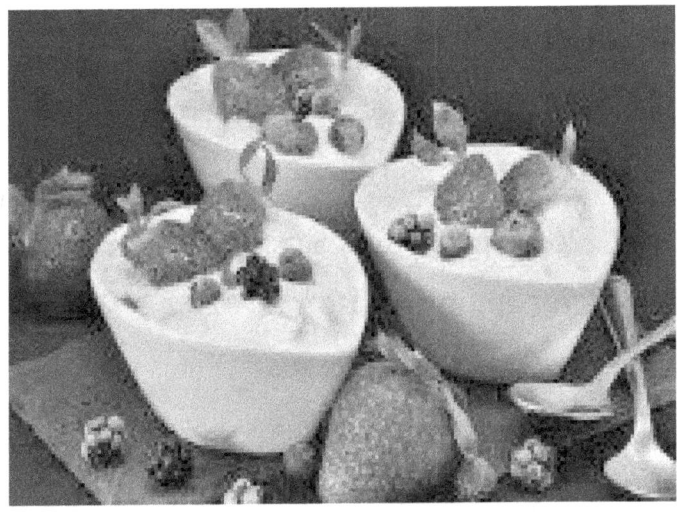

Find yourself a tasty ketogenic treat in this segment that is fit for a king or queen!

Brownie Muffins

Serving Yields: 6

Macros: 4.4 g Net Carbs | 183 Calories| 7 g Protein |13 g Total Fats

Fixings Needed:

- Salt - .5 tsp.
- Flaxseed meal – 1 cup
- Cocoa powder - .25 cup
- Cinnamon – 1 tbsp.
- Baking powder - .5 tbsp.
- Coconut oil – 2 tbsp.
- Large egg - 1
- Vanilla extract – 1 tsp.
- Sugar-free caramel syrup - .25 cup
- Pumpkin puree - .5 cup
- Slivered almonds - .5 cup
- Apple cider vinegar – 1 tsp.

How to Prepare:

1. Set the oven temperature to 350°F.
2. Use a deep mixing container — mix all of the fixings and stir well.
3. Use 6 paper liners in the muffin tin and add 1/4 cup of batter to each one.
4. Sprinkle several almonds on the tops, pressing gently.
5. Bake approximately 15 minutes or when the top is set.

Meal Prep Tips:

1. Cut the brownies into six portions.
2. Store in plastic baggies for the fridge or freezer bags if you want to have them last longer than 3-4 days.

Cheesecake Cupcakes

Serving Yields: 12

Macros: 2.1 g Net Carbs | 204 Calories| 5 g Protein | 20 g Total Fats

Fixings Needed:

- Almond meal – .5 cup
- Melted butter – .25 cup
- Eggs – 2
- Softened cream cheese – 2 – 8 oz. pkg.
- Stevia or your favorite sweetener – .75 cup
- Vanilla extract – 1 tsp.

How to Prepare:

1. Warm up the oven until it reaches 350ºF. Prepare a muffin tin with 12 paper liners.

2. Combine the butter and almond meal. Spoon into the cups to make a flat crust.
3. Whisk the vanilla, sweetener of choice, eggs, and cream cheese with an electric mixer until creamy. Scoop it in on top of the crust.
4. Bake for 15-17 minutes.

Meal Prep Tips:

1. Once they're done the cooking cycle, just remove and cool at room temperature.
2. You can store them overnight or at least 8 hours in the fridge.
3. Enjoy anytime for a delicious treat.

Cinnamon Apples – Instant Pot

Serving Yields: 4 large dishes

Macros: 2 g Net Carbs |110 Calories| 9 g Protein | 3 g Total Fats

Fixings Needed:

- Brown sugar - .5 cup - keto-friendly substitute
- Sugar - .5 cup or Swerve – 2 tsp.
- Cinnamon – 1 tbsp.
- Nutmeg - .125 tsp.
- Unsalted butter – 2 tbsp.
- Cornstarch – 3 tbsp.
- Granny Smith apples – 6
- Salt – 1 pinch

How to Prepare:

1. Peel and slice the apples thin.
2. Combine all of the fixings in the Instant Pot. Press the manual function for 18 minutes. Natural release the pressure (10 min.) and open the pot.
3. Stir and serve or prep.
4. Note: The macro totals are calculated using regular sugar and brown sugar.

Meal Prep Tips:

1. Let the apples cool to room temperature. Store in an airtight container or heavy-duty freezer bags.
2. Refrigerate for up to 7 days.
3. You can keep the apples fresh in the freezer for about 2 months.

Delicious No-Bake Coconut Cookies

Serving Yields: 20

Macros: -0- g Net Carbs | 99 Calories| 3 g Protein |10 g Total Fats

Fixings Needed:

- Melted coconut oil – 1 cup
- Monk fruit sweetened maple syrup or sweetener of choice - .5 cup
- Shredded unsweetened coconut flakes – 3 cups

How to Prepare:

1. Cut out a sheet of parchment paper and place on a cookie tray.

2. Combine all of the fixings. Run your hands through some water from the tap and shape the mixture into small balls. Arrange them on the pan around one to two inches apart.
3. Press them down to form a cookie and refrigerate until firm.

Meal Prep Tips:

1. You can prepare these into individual bags if you're an on-the-go kind of person.
2. The cookies will remain fresh covered for up to 7 days at room temperature.
3. Store in the fridge for up to a month.
4. If you choose, you can freeze the cookies for up to two months.

Mocha Cheesecake Bars

Serving Yields: 16

Macros: 3 g Net Carbs | 232 Calories| 6 g Protein | 21 g Total Fats

Fixings Needed for the Brownie Layer

- Vanilla extract – 2 tsp.
- Unsalted butter – 6 tbsp.
- Large eggs - 3
- Almond flour – 1.5 cups
- Hershey's Baking Cocoa - .5 cup
- Erythritol – 1 cup
- Salt - .5 tsp.
- Instant coffee - .5 tbsp.
- Baking powder – 1 tsp.

Fixings Needed for the Cream Cheese Layer

- Erythritol - .5 cup
- Softened cream cheese – 1 lb.
- Large egg - 1
- Vanilla extract – 1 tsp
- Also Needed: 8x8-inch baking pan

How to Prepare:

1. Warm up the oven to 350°F. Lightly grease or spray the pan with a spritz or oil cooking spray.
2. Combine the wet fixings starting with the vanilla and butter and mix in the eggs.
3. In another container, combine the dry ingredients and whisk with the wet fixings. Set aside 1/4 cup of the batter for later. Pour the mixture into the pan.

4. Mix the cream cheese (room temperature) with the rest of the ingredients for the second layer. Spread it on the layer of brownies.
5. Use the reserved batter as the last layer (will be thin). Bake 30-35 minutes.

Meal Prep Tips:

1. When cooled, slice the cheesecake bars.
2. Store in the fridge for several days or freeze in containers or freezer bags for extended use. Be sure to date and add the name of the contents.

Peanut Butter Fudge

Serving Yields: 18

Macros: -0- g Net Carbs |89 Calories| 2 g Protein | 8 g Total Fats

Fixings Needed:

- Peanut butter - .5 cup
- Coconut oil - .5 cup
- Sweetener of choice – ex. liquid stevia granulated sweetener – to taste
- Also Needed: 12-18 count muffin tin & liners or a loaf pan

How to Prepare:

1. Prepare the tin of choice with some cooking spray or a spritz of oil.
2. Combine the oil and peanut butter together on the stovetop or microwave. Melt and add the sweetener.

Meal Prep Tips:

1. Scoop the mixture into the tins or loaf pan and freeze.
2. You can serve with some (optional) melted chocolate – but count the carbs. Enjoy your treat anytime.

Spice Cakes

Serving Yields: 12

Macros: 3 g Net Carbs | 277 Calories| 6 g Protein | 27 g Total Fats

Fixings Needed:

- Eggs - 4
- Baking powder – 2 tsp.
- Almond flour – 2 cups
- Salted butter - .5 cup
- Nutmeg - .5 tsp.
- Allspice - .5 tsp.
- Ginger - .5 tsp.
- Cinnamon - .5 tsp
- Erythritol - .75 cup
- Ground cloves - .25 tsp.
- Vanilla extract – 1 tsp.
- Water – 5 tbsp.

How to Prepare:

1. Set the temperature in the oven to 350°F. Prepare a cupcake tray with liners (12).

2. Mix the butter and erythritol with a hand mixer. Once it's smooth, combine with 2 eggs and the vanilla. Mix and stir in the remainder of the eggs, stirring until creamy.

3. Grind the clove to a fine powder and add with the rest of the spices. Whisk into the mixture. Stir in the baking powder and almond flour. Blend in the water. When the batter is smooth, add to the prepared tin.

4. Bake for 15 minutes. Enjoy any time.

Meal Prep Tips:

1. Cool thoroughly for the prep.
2. Store in the fridge for a few days or in the freezer to enjoy later.
3. Be sure to label it with the date and its contents accurately.

Vanilla Cinnamon Protein Bites

Serving Yields: 18-20 bites

Macros: 4 g Net Carbs |112 Calories| 2 g Protein | 9 g Total Fats

Fixings Needed:

- Nut butter of choice - .25 - .33 cup
- Pure maple syrup - .25 - .33 cup
- Protein powder – vanilla - .25 cup
- Almond meal - .5 cup
- Vanilla extract - .5 – 1 tsp.
- Quick oats - .75 cup
- Cinnamon – 1 tbsp.
- Also Needed: Food processor

How to Prepare:

1. Line a cookie tin with a layer of parchment paper.
2. Grind the oats with the processor and add to a mixing container. Combine the cinnamon, protein powder, almond meal, and nut butter.
3. Mix in the syrup and vanilla. Using your hands, mix well and roll into small balls.
4. Freeze for 20-30 minutes.
5. Arrange in a Ziplock-type baggie with the cinnamon and vanilla protein.

Meal Prep Tips:

1. After dusting the bites, store in the fridge for three weeks.
2. Store in the freezer for up to six months.

Chapter 10:

<u>A Final Recommendation</u>

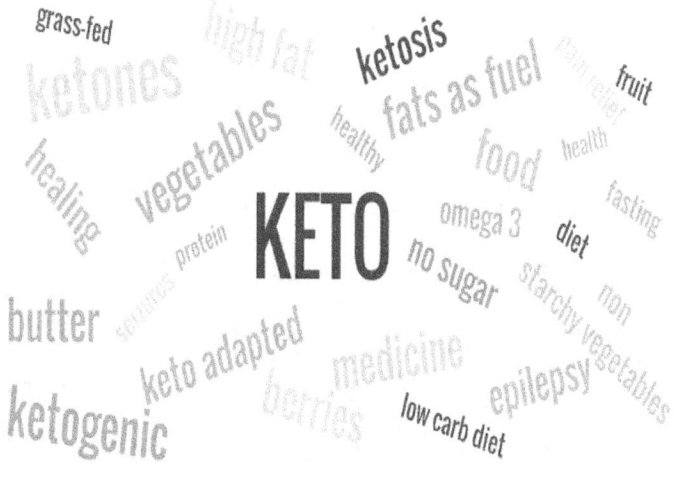

The preparation for a ketogenic diet doesn't have to be a commitment of time nor excessive resources. The same thing shouldn't take away the pleasure of being at the table. Simply, adapt to a ketogenic lifestyle without sacrificing your freedom.

How to Avoid Meal Prep Mistakes Using Keto

Limit psychological & physical stress during evening hours: It is essential for you to recharge and take the evening hours to relax and improve your sleep hygiene. Try to leave work – at work. Deal with the issues in the morning. If you are going through a tough time or working long hours, you tend to forget items you may 'munch' on as you are working. Make it a point to write down everything you eat.

Working long hours can be beneficial for knocking off those pounds, but it can also cause you to be restless and can lead to post-workout insomnia if you have worked out or done other strenuous physical activities on your evenings off.

No matter what the case, slow down for at least an hour or more before attempting to retire for the evening.

Expect plateaus with your weight loss plan: If you have dieted before, you already know you will reach spans of time where your weight loss will level out. That's merely a segment of weight loss that can't be moderated. All you need to do is remain consistent. The weight loss will return. It is much better to expect problems or roadblocks than it is to believe new dieting methods or fasting (if you choose) will be smooth sailing. Be sure you have selected a time where your social events will not interfere with your dieting plan selected.

Reassess & adjust your goals as needed: After you have adjusted your body to the ketogenic dieting plan, you can start using an intermittent fasting method if you choose to take that route. Be willing to change your goals as you make progress. By starting small, you leave the door open so you can make more significant challenges as you proceed through the plan.

Use Free Apps

You'll need to keep track of the exact amount of protein, net carbs, and total fat that you eat every day. Research has shown individuals who keep records of their food activity will more than likely be successful with weight loss. You will always be able to move forward when you discover any weaknesses that exist in your dieting success.

My Food Diary: Occasionally, you may need to look up nutritional facts to ensure you have the correct carbohydrate, protein, and fats in your diet plan.

Standard Keto Calculator: You will achieve the perfect mixture of the traditional keto diet plan of 5% carbs, 25% protein, and 70% ratios. (This is a general ratio.)

MyFitnessPal has been chosen as one of the best apps available to track your macros as rated by Consumer Reports and PC Magazine's Editor's Choice Selection. It's free to download, but you can also choose to update to a premium plan for higher rates.

Check Units of Measurement: Many of the recipes you will discover over the Internet or other sources may be listed in Imperial (ex. pounds) or in the Metric system.

Seek Group Support & Don't Diet Alone: Try dieting with a friend or coworker to make the challenge more interesting. With everyone on the same page, you can better plan a delicious meal. However, everyone may enjoy the changes after the initial advances. Research and locate a support group in your area. Praise others for all accomplishments.

<u>Last But Not Least - Practice Mindful Eating:</u> It is vital to take a few extra moments to enjoy the flavors and textures of your food. The ketogenic diet will provide all of the nourishment to remain successful dieting. Enjoy your time spent with the conversation of a friend or family member. Drink your water and sip your tea or coffee. Feel satisfied and enjoy the moment. Stop rushing around at dinner time.

Make Traveling Using Keto Effortless

Enjoy a low-carbohydrate breakfast before you travel consisting of cooked bacon, hard-boiled eggs, plain Greek yogurt with berries, or nuts and cream. Warm up some egg muffins for a quick pick-me-up. If you have a few extra minutes, slice an avocado or saute some mushrooms and sausage with tomatoes; just give the mixture a splash of olive oil or keto-friendly mayo. If you will be traveling in the car try some of these snacks:

- Homemade salad
- Raw green veggies (+) dip
- Hard-boiled eggs
- Meat or cheese packs
- Canned or packages of tuna

On your journey, the 'worst case scenario' happens and you do not see an eatery anywhere in sight. Look for a grocery or convenience store. Even the smallest country stores will probably stock part of these items:

- Almonds
- Hard-boiled eggs
- Deli meat
- String cheese
- Pork rinds

Have Appropriate Containers for Traveling

Consider making a 'run-away' bag of essential items to maintain ketosis while you are living your busy lifestyle. These are a few:

- For bacon – A new toothbrush case – (It can be cheap and discard after it's used.)
- For butter: Pack a new soap case.
- For olive oil: pack a 4-oz. leak-proof bottle
- For mayo or home-made nut butter: 1 high-quality squeezable bottle
- For cream cheese, dip, nuts, etc.: 1 medium container
- For veggies, dip, etc.: A refrigerated container

You can also use the same containers used for meal prep in your kitchen.

Conclusion

I hope you have enjoyed your new experience with meal prep using the Keto **Meal Prep Cookbook:** Beginner Ketogenic Diet For Weight-Loss With Low-Carb Food. Hopefully, you have found many new ways to prepare meals for you and your family. I would like to provide you with a few ideas to carry with you as you proceed using meal prep and your ketogenic techniques for dieting.

- Think long-term of how keto will work for you.
- Keep your intake of carbs low.
- Prepare a food journal and familiarize yourself with an online app to remain in ketosis with ease.

- Gather a food list of your favorite spices and other products to convert your pantry to keto.
- Begin using your new diet plan, remembering you can adjust the menu plan using the carbohydrate limitations you have each day.

You have all of the tools to be successful, but you still need to understand how to test to ensure you are in ketosis. Your individual progress can be tested using several items to ensure you remain in a ketogenic state. They include testing your breath, blood, or urine.

Take a blood test. It is recommended by the American Diabetes Association to test your blood using the blood ketone meter, particularly during times you are ill. Add a small drop of blood on a testing strip and insert the tab into the meter. It will indicate the amount of beta-hydroxybutyrate in your bloodstream. The results are highly accurate and consistent. Unfortunately, the strips are expensive and if you are squeamish of needles, this is not for you.

Test your breath. A Ketonix meter will provide you with a way to test your breath for ketosis. You just breathe into the meter to receive a special coded color. You will compare those colors with a guideline strip provided in the package. It is less messy, but it does take longer to get a reading.

Test your urine. One huge advantage of testing our urine is that the strips are inexpensive and can detect acetoacetate - one of the ketone bodies. The strip is dipped into the urine which will change the color of the strip. The various shades of purple and pink will clearly indicate the levels of the ketones.

The darker the color on the testing strip, the higher the level of ketones. Early morning testing provides the most accurate score after a ketogenic diet dinner the evening before testing.

However, long-term testing with the strips is not as accurate as other methods. It can be misleading since the acetoacetate will only show up if they are in excessive levels. As your body adapts to ketosis, it will use the acetoacetate and the levels would read lower even if you're in ketosis.

There is no time like the present to gather your lists of goods needed to begin your ketogenic way of living. Begin with your food and prep items and before you know it, you will be prepping your freezer to the maximum with all the delicious keto foods your body is craving.

If you have a few moments, I would appreciate a review on Amazon if you found your new book useful in any way.

Enjoy your new way of living!

www.ingramcontent.com/pod-product-compliance
Lightning Source LLC
Chambersburg PA
CBHW071245220526
45468CB00001B/5